Spiritual Guides

to

HOLISTIC HEALTH

and HAPPINESS

Robert E. Valett

Poppy Lane Publishing Co.
Fresno, CA

Published and distributed in the United States by
Poppy Lane Publishing Company
5308 N. Colonial #102, Fresno, CA 93704
(209)449-9067

Valett, Robert E.
Spirtual Guides to Holistic Health and Happiness
Includes bibliographical references
ISBN: 0-938911-11-2
1. Spirituality 2. Holistic Health 3. Happiness

Artistic designs by the author

Printed by CAL VALLEY PRINTING
Madera, California

This book presents helpful insights on how to obtain holistic health and happiness, as advocated by many great spiritual guides including:

Aristotle, Matthew Arnold, Maya Angelou, Marcus Aurelius, Francis Bacon, Tegh Bahadur, Ludwig van Beethoven, Robert Browning, Gautama Buddha, George Burns, Jesus Christ, Winston Churchill, Confucius, Norman Cousins, Democritus, Emily Dickinson, Larry Dossey, Fyodor Dostoyevski, J.B. Downie, John Dryden, Thomas Edison, Albert Einstein, Loren Eisely, Ralph Waldo Emerson, Epictetus, William Faulkner, Benjamin Franklin, Spencer Michael Free, Kahlil Gibran, Johann Wolfgang von Goethe, Edgar A. Guest, Nick Herbert, Thich Nhat Hanh, Langston Hughes, Victor Hugo, Hippocrates, William James, Thomas Jefferson, Carl Jung, John Keats, Omar Khayyam, Soren Kierkegaard, Abraham Lincoln, Henry Wadsworth Longfellow, James Madison, Rollo May, Katherine Mansfield, Edna St. Vincent Millay, John Milton, Seneca, William Shakespeare, Sir Walter Scott, Percy Bysshe Shelley, King Solomon, St. Francis of Assisi, Benedict Spinoza, Alfred Lord Tennyson, Norman Thomas, Henry David Thoreau, Mark Twain, Lao Tzu, Izaak Walton, Walt Whitman, William Wordsworth, Erwin Schrodinger, Ogden Nash, Reinhold Niebuhr, Mary Oliver, Alexander Pope, Pythagoras, Adrienne Rich, Eleanor Roosevelt, Franklin D. Roosevelt, Rabindrarath Tagore, Mother Teresa, and others.

Jesus said

Thou shalt love the Lord thy God
with all thy heart,
and with all thy soul,
and with all thy mind,
and with all thy strength:
this is the first commandment.
And the second is:
Love thy neighbor as thyself.
-Mark 12:30-31

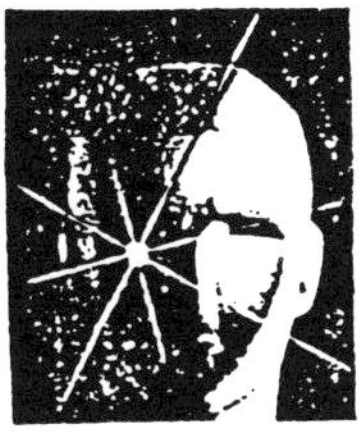

- Dedication -

This book is dedicated to Norman Cousins and the many kindred souls who have taught that the human spirit is the single most identifiable feature of human experience - and unless it is understood and respected, all other facts are secondary.

- Acknowledgements -

I wish to acknowledge my major spiritual mentors, Norman Cousins, Ralph Waldo Emerson, Benjamin Franklin, Carl G. Jung, M.D. and Mark Twain, whose unique contributions to humankind have motivated me to write this book. Thanks to Paul Adams, Roberta and Ian Bell, Helen Bellman, Doris Dillon, Jane Fischer, Dr. Nancy Hunt, Dr. Susan Shanks, Shirley Valett, Jack Welch, M.D. and Phyllis and Wendell Wilson for their time and effort in reading and commenting on the manuscript.

Recognition is also due to Argus Communications, P.O. Box 6000, Allen Texas 75002, for prior publication of my motivational posters as marked with an asterisk (*) within this book. Those compositions not credited in this work are my own.

I am especially grateful for the interest and suggestions received from students in my classes at California State University, Fresno and from participants in my early workshops at the Fresno, California Retired Teachers Association. Appreciation is also expressed for the ongoing feedback received from participants in my various holistic health, creative meditation and positive thinking presentations.

Special acknowledgment must be expressed to Myrna Bolger and other staff members and patients who participated in my holistic health and mental imagery presentations through the Humor and Music program at St. Agnes Hospital, Fresno, California. Similarly, the staff at the Valley Children's Hospital in Fresno has been very supportive of my ongoing participation with my dog in their pet therapy program. Without the inspirational help from all these persons, this work would not have been possible.

Robert E. Valett

- CONTENTS -

- Personal Principles Of Holistic Health And Happiness -

1. Actively pursue happiness with a healthy life style.

2. Understand that happiness and good health are holistic states of well-being resulting from a harmonious interaction between your spirit, soul, mind and body.

3. Acknowledge that all persons are interdependent beings in need of physical and spiritual help and guidance.

4. Believe that loving care of self, others and the global community is the most powerful spiritual force in your life.

5. Through prayer and meditation, open your self and relate to the higher spiritual and universal forces of which you are an important part.

6. Constructively affirm your personal strengths, goals and aspirations.

7. Laugh and be well by learning from humorous situations, inappropriate actions and your own stupid mistakes.

8. Clearly imagine what you would like to become and how this vision might be realized.

9. Express your unique creative spirit, talents and abilities.

10. Nurture the healing force within you.

11. Know and esteem yourself, exert self-discipline and assume self and social responsibility.

12. Work cooperatively for the common good and a better world.

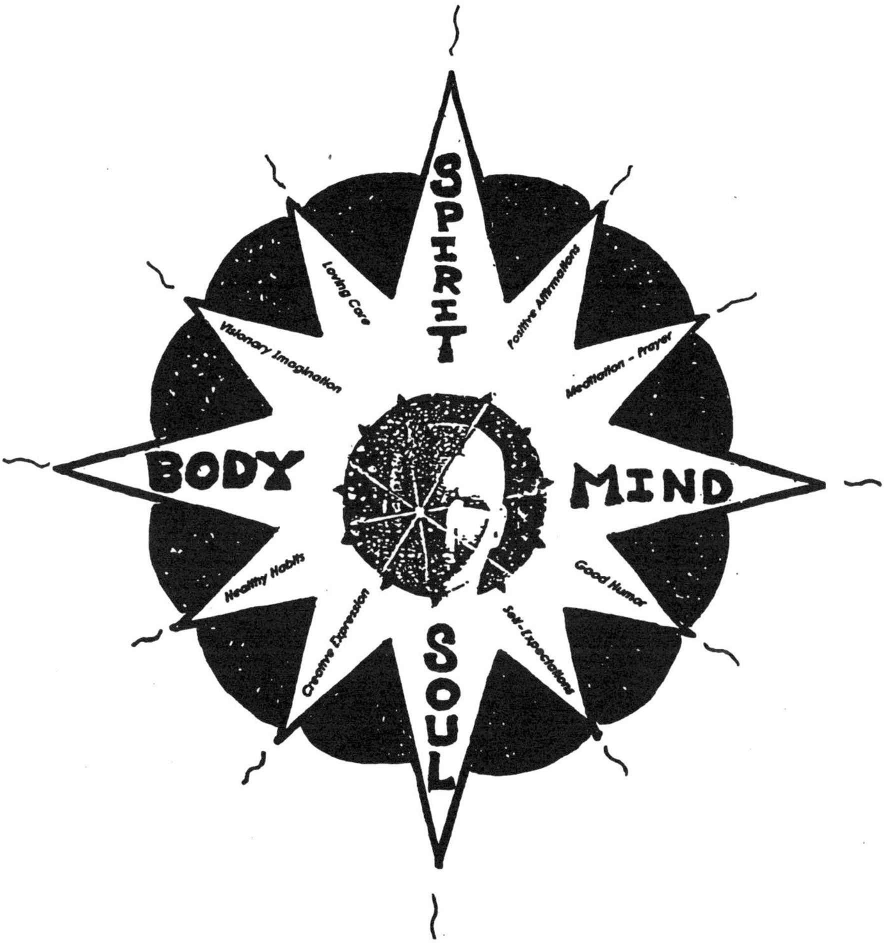

Vital Spiritual Forces

PREFACE

By our own spirits are we deified
-William Wordsworth

This book presents spiritual wisdom and insights which can guide us to holistic health and happiness. We are all possessed by spirits which guide us through our daily lives. All living things consist of dynamic spiritual elements which arouse them to action. These spirits are inherent in the unique souls of all persons, are awakened by their minds and expressed through their heartfelt emotions and behavior.

Humankind is a unique life form activated by invisible spiritual elements and shaped by mysterious cosmic energies and quantum forces. In order to live happy and fruitful lives, we must nurture the vital spirits of life within us and attempt to understand the nature of these powers and how they might best be utilized. Through the balanced integration of spirit, soul, body and mind we can achieve healthy and happy states of being.

Spirit is the essential immaterial breath of life which ignites our deepest feelings and intuitions and refines our thoughts and actions. Our vital spirits are reflected in a personal sense of energy, vitality and healthfulness which makes it possible to engage the challenges of life in constructive and creative ways. A person in good spirits also displays enthusiasm, zest and joy in living.

Developing our vital spirits enables us to better cope with the difficult tasks of human survival and self-realization. The divine nature of humanity gleams forth through positive expressions of spiritual potentialities - such as love, humor, music and other attributes of a civilized community. Our unique spiritual gifts enable us to live a more joyful and happy life.

The major challenge of human beings is to consciously and purposely channel our creative spirits - and to properly manage our destructive inclinations. Human spirits are both creatively good and destructively bad. Frequently we feel in "good spirits", and are overjoyed by the renewing spirits of life such as love, creative expression, fun and celebration which result in much happiness. But occasionally we feel in "bad spirits", seemingly possessed by anger, hate, hopelessness and fear which drive us to increasing despair and violence.

Life itself consists of creative spirits ever moving onward in the perpetual adaptation and generation of novel possibilities. Through gradual evolutionary change, humankind has finally developed to the point of conscious participation in the actual realization of its potentialities. We are all spiritual beings involved in the never ending choice and development of whatever we willfully decide to become! And our spiritual forces are released and channeled through deliberate choice and responsible action.

A conscious decision is often a major step to do something that will *in*spire us to creatively enrich our lives. And we are personally responsible for selectively "tuning into" those spirits of life that we wish to guide us. Successful human development depends on our adaptation to cultural and environmental changes through never ending *conscious choice and adjustment* to the consequences of our thoughts and actions.

We can kindle when we will
the fire which in the heart resides,
the spirit bloweth and is still,
in mystery our soul abides:
But tasks in hours of insight will'd
can be through hours of gloom fulfill'd
-Matthew Arnold

We actually become self-creative beings by building our lives through an integral process involving spirit, thought and action. Like newly apprenticed stone masons, we may be awkward in our first efforts at self-construction. Or with time and effort we may progress to the journeyman stage of skillful development. But hopefully, we are all challenged by the possibilities of becoming even more proficient in erecting our own glorious cathedrals to the human spirit, mind and body.

Our dreams, choices and willful striving all help determine whatever bodily or other physical form the cathedrals we have designed may take in reality. But eventually, our vital spirits assume some form of physical reality through the holistic efforts of body, mind and soul. Inner harmony is essential for personal health, success and happiness. And it is the uniquely energizing spirits of harmonious body, mind and soul which bring joy and distinguish one's creative endeavors.

According to extensive surveys, conducted by George Gallup pollsters over a fifty year period of time, we are a very spiritual people. More than 95 percent of Americans say they believe in God and pray regularly and 40 percent of those polled report "unusual, life-changing" spiritual experiences. Interestingly, people who profess to "spiritual experiences" tend to change their lives toward a more ethical and socially responsible direction.

The pollsters also found that highly spiritual people derive more meaning from life, are far happier than the rest of the population, are more tolerant and eager to reach out to others and are more involved in charitable activities. Surprisingly, this kind of spirituality has little to do with church affiliation or attendance. However, the great majority of Americans do feel that religion is very important in their lives. But most people in all cultures and times have been highly spiritual beings regardless of religious denomination.

Happiness resides not in possessions
and not in gold,
the feeling of happiness dwells in the soul.
-Democritus

From the very beginning of history, mankind has been in awe of great and mysterious powers beyond its comprehension. With the gradual acquisition of knowledge and scientific methodology, we are now increasingly capable of understanding more about the universal elements which affect human behavior - including our own potentialities for self-realization. But our inherent limitations of evolutionary time and development make it impossible to ever fully comprehend or control the vast cosmic powers within and about us. Even so, through holistic efforts of our bodies, minds and spirits, we have become active co-creators of the world in which we live.

With increasing population and other social, economic and environmental problems, people have become increasingly subject to the stresses of personal and social failure. At times, it seems that the world is engulfed in the self-made misery of ignorant and destructively evil men and women. In many places traditional values and institutions such as the family, school, church and community have become more dysfunctional with rising crime, health problems and personal concerns.

I myself am Heaven or Hell.
-Omar Khayyam

At the same time, many individuals have experienced a profound loss of faith in themselves and their governmental institutions and cannot adequately cope with these problems. In times of trial and self-wrenching turmoil, it is good to test alternative solutions to our problems. Wise men and women have long recognized the remarkable regenerative powers of spirit, soul, mind and body; these insights and discoveries have been recorded in the great literature and records of many cultures and serve as powerful spiritual guides to all concerned.

Much of this wisdom has recently been validated and extended through modern scientific research and clinical practice. Accordingly, we have significantly increased our understanding of these human powers and how they might be used in our personal quests for self- realization. Now we have insightful knowledge available to help us make wise and responsible choices as to how we can successfully continue our pursuits of happiness.

Self-empowerment and determination is crucial in human affairs. It is only through the continued expansion of self-control, knowledge and realization of our special potentialities in a supportive community that we can really become successful and happy persons. Indeed, personal happiness and the fate of humankind and the planet earth all depend on the enlightenment of the human soul and the nurturance of the vast creative powers within one's Self.

Give birth again to the dream...Lift up your hearts-
Each new hour holds new chances for new beginnings.
-Maya Angelou

Spiritual guides are invaluable sources of inspiration. These guides are available to us through the model lives and teaching of religious leaders such as Buddha, Moses, Jesus, Mohammed, Gandhi, the Dali Lama, Mother Teresa and numerous other contemporary "good Samaritans" in every community. Some spiritual guides may be recognized in the more secular lives of great humanitarian statespersons (Thomas Jefferson, Eleanor Roosevelt, Ralph Bunche, Jimmy Carter and others) - and even highly ethical businessmen devoted to the betterment of their workers and communities. Another source of spiritual guidance is to be found in the grand works of many poets, musicians, artists, and philosophers who may appear to have angelic-like qualities worthy of devotion and emulation.

This book presents a summarization of wisdom of the sages that has been found inspirationally helpful to many persons by enabling them to understand and employ their own vital spirits of life and happiness. The star-like geometric design on the page preceding this preface portrays the human image in the symbolic process of becoming self-realized. Self-realization is a dynamic holistic process that requires a relatively balanced integration of spirit, mind, body and soul as represented by the four major directional beams. Several relatively minor powers of self-determination are represented by the eight shorter star-like rays of the design including loving care, visionary imagination, healthy habits, creative expression, self-expectations, good humor, prayerful meditation and positive affirmations. Each of these vital spirits is discussed and illustrated in the book with quotations and comments by widely esteemed personages.

The first chapter presents an overview of the basic significance of happiness in human affairs and how it is attained. This is followed by chapters on all twelve of the vital spiritual forces involved in the process of holistic health and self-realization as listed above and as portrayed by emanating star beams in the design. The last two chapters discuss the celebration of community and human spiritual evolution as culminating steps in the pursuit of happiness - for it is only through the continued development of human fellowship that we are able to survive and flourish.

Very important parts of the book are the "personal surveys" for reader response and involvement, which are placed at the end of each chapter. Survey responses can also be used as discussion points with friends to stimulate further personal insight and understanding. A brief supplement of related thoughts for personal reflection and meditation is provided at the end of the book along with some blank pages for use as needed.

Hopefully, the ideas presented in this book will inspire the reader to further consideration and contemplation of the works and teachings of these and other spiritual guides, who can help to create a more wholesome and joyful life. Any application of the wisdom presented by these guides is bound to contribute to personal growth and happiness!

Today, well lived, makes every yesterday a dream of happiness and every tomorrow a vision of hope.
-From the Sanskrit

1

---- HAPPINESS---

There is nothing better than to be happy, to rejoice, and to do good in life.
-Ecclesiastes 3:12

Happiness is an emotional feeling of great pleasure, contentment, gladness and joy which people in all times and places have struggled to achieve. The ancient Hindu text, *Bhagavad-Gita*, declared that happiness is the universal aim in life. In the book of *Ecclesiastes*, Biblical preachers proclaimed that there is nothing better than happiness and joy in human life. The great philosopher, *Aristotle*, avowed that happiness is the meaning and the purpose of life, the whole aim and end of human existence.

There are numerous things in life that make people happy, such as feeling the first rays of sunshine on a cold and misty morning, the touch of a loved one or when a person feels good about something he or she has done. Marcus Aurelius believed that very little is actually needed to make a happy life since happiness is an internal state largely determined by our way of thinking. What we actually think and believe determines how we act and what we might do to achieve happiness.

It is important to feel good and happy about ourselves, our relationships with others and the world in which we live. The happy person has learned that the first passion of the human soul is joy in living. But joyful living results from the achievement and celebration of meaningful, self-fulfilling experiences, such as love, friendship and creative endeavor. Bertrand Russell was another great reflective thinker who concluded that wide interests and affection for other people are what most bring zest and joy in life - which is the essence of happiness.

The American Declaration of Independence does acknowledge that all persons have been endowed by their Creator with certain unalienable rights and that among these are life, liberty, and the pursuit of happiness. But Thomas Jefferson wrote that, although we have the right to pursue happiness, its actual attainment depends on our personal goals and responsible actions. It is only when happiness is individually contemplated, understood and courageously pursued that it is realized.

Happiness is a form of courage.
-Holbrook Jackson

One's personal pursuit of happiness is a lifelong quest for pleasure and satisfaction. But happiness is a relative and transitory state of mind and being, which results from the momentary attainment of what a person considers to be good and valuable at the time. Happiness constantly comes and goes. Even so, according to scientific surveys, most people claim to be happy with their lives much of the time.

These studies have also disclosed the major factors involved in becoming happy. For example, people who are frequently involved in a variety of enjoyable experiences report themselves as being happy. Happy persons also tend to remember more of their good experiences than unhappy ones. Good self-esteem and satisfaction with life events, such as job contentment, are also very important components of happiness.

Most people are about as happy as they make up their minds to be.
-Abraham Lincoln

We constantly define and creatively build our own happiness from day to day by what we think and do. The starting point is to decide what we want to do that will make us happy. People who increase their regular participation in favored activities become happier. Those who spend time doing new and novel things also have a greater sense of joy and well-being. Purposeful goals with challenging activities that are intrinsically rewarding are most pleasurable and satisfying. Some of the most common activities that frequently result in happiness are:

Being with friends
Having a lively talk
Laughing
Listening to music
Doing a job well
Enjoying exercise
Sleeping soundly
Helping others
Creating something
Gardening
Reflecting on "good times"
Having new experiences
Reading
Being told one is loved
Expressing love to someone
Seeing beautiful scenery
Being relaxed
Being with animals
Having fun with leisure time activities
Praying & meditating
Making positive self-assertions
Volunteering
Achieving reasonable goals
Traveling
Delighting in food & refreshment
Developing a new skill or ability

The creative pursuit of happiness requires self-understanding, personal goals and persistent effort. It assumes that whatever happiness is realized will be the result of constructive encounters and experiences with self and others. Studies actually show that persons with a framework of values or philosophy that provides meaning to their lives report greater happiness; these individuals also prove to be more successful, more charitable and more concerned with helping to create a just or better world. The amount or degree of happiness that a person experiences can be significantly increased through conscious decisions to practice appropriate values and behaviors.

It is probably a mistake to pursue happiness;
much better to create happiness;
still better to create happiness for others.
The more happiness you create for others
the more will be yours.
-Lloyd Douglas

Although our values and deliberate actions are major factors in determining how successful our pursuit of happiness will be, there are a number of limiting circumstances to be considered. For instance, some evidence exists that a genetic predisposition for unhappiness, sadness and grief runs in families and at times may be severe enough to require medical treatment. The sources of happiness also vary between the sexes with women usually deriving primary satisfaction from children and family, while most men gain more pleasure from business and political affairs.

Loving relationships are more productive of happiness for all people. Married men and women consistently report being happier than people who are divorced, widowed or otherwise single. Optimists are generally happier than pessimists. Loneliness is strongly associated with unhappiness and single men tend to be the least happy.

Moods of happiness are associated with states of rest and relaxation. Appropriate exercise stimulates a sense of healthy well-being. When cognitive activity is minimized during prayer or meditation, the feeling of happiness and contentment is greatly enhanced; people who talk to others and are socially involved also tend to be happier than those who are not.

Life is a gift, life is happiness,
each moment can be an age of happiness.
-Fyodor Dostoyevski

Age and time are other important factors to consider. Significantly more persons over age 65 report being pleased with their lives than those between 18 and 49. For people under 35, women are more happy than men, while for those over 55 years of age, men are happier than women. Parents under age 50 are less happy (especially those with adolescents) than non-parents, but over age 50 there is no difference between those who have adult children and those who do not have children. In many respects family life is the source of most happiness and unhappiness!

There is no escape in life from the sadness of loss, failure or rejection. Happiness only has meaning when it is balanced by some degree of unhappiness which all persons are bound to experience. Hopefully, we can profit from our personal sorrows and tragedies by becoming more complete and capable in dealing with future problems. And our memories of good and happy times can always help us renew our spirit of life to cope with the morrow.

Happiness is attained through balanced and harmonious experiences of our body, mind, spirit and soul. Some of the more successful experiences which result in happiness are discussed in the rest of this book. These include loving care, positive affirmation, visionary imagination, meditation and prayer, healthy habits, good humor, creative expression and reasonable self-expectations.

Most often, the successful pursuit of happiness depends on realistic goals and plans for achieving them. And the attainment of individual aspirations invariably involves many other people. By actively engaging in appropriate experiences with others, we can help create a joyful community and more fully realize personal happiness!

Happy the man, and happy he alone, who can call today his own.
He who, secure within, can say:
tomorrow do thy worst, for I have lived today.
-John Dryden

+++HAPPINESS+++

He builded his happiness out of these:
Birds and blossoms and friendly trees,
Books that stood on a little shelf,
Three or four neighbors, much like himself,
The wife and children who bore his name
And he asked no favors from wealth or fame.

He found delight in his garden plot,
Knew marigold and forget-me-not;
He walked the hills, and he fished the streams,
With friends he trusted he shared his dreams.
He was sometimes merry and sometimes sad,
But he made the most of what joys he had.

He found his thrills in the lesser things.
The joy a blossoming peony brings;
The merry songs and the kindly mirth
Of the gentle women and men of earth
He thanked his God for the right to live,
And he never asked more than life could give.

Seekers for happiness wander far,
And, oh, how jaded and tired they are,
Forever pursuing the strange new thrill
They never have caught and never will!
But he found friendship and flowers and trees,
And builded his happiness out of these.

-Edgar A. Guest

*-The ABC's of Happiness-

ASPIRE to realize your potential

BELIEVE in yourself

CREATE a good life

DREAM about what you might become

EXERCISE frequently

FORGIVE honest mistakes

GLORIFY the creative spirit

HUMOR yourself and others

IMAGINE great things

JOYFULLY live each day

KINDLY help others

LOVE one another

MEDITATE daily

NURTURE the environment

ORGANIZE for harmonious action

PRAISE performance well done

QUESTION most things

REGULATE your own behavior

SMILE often

THINK rationally

UNDERSTAND yourself

VALUE life

WORK for the common good

X-RAY and carefully examine problems

YEARN to improve

ZESTFULLY pursue happiness

- A Personal Happiness Survey -

This is the time to stop and reflect on your own life and happiness by completing the following sentences as rapidly as you can. Express the first thought or feeling that comes to your mind. Make additional comments as needed.

1. Some of the things I really enjoy doing are-

2. My primary goal in life is-

3. My major talents include-

4. I have been quite successful at-

5. What I value most is-

6. When I was a child I most enjoyed-

7. What really makes me happy is-

8. What makes me unhappy is-

9. One of the most happy times in my life was-

10. I believe I could become more happy by-

2

---- SPIRIT ----

God is spirit, and those who worship him must worship him in spirit and truth.
-John 4:24

The spirit of life is infused in you at conception. It is the vigorous essence in life that springs from the cosmic spark which created your unique human soul. From this beginning, your spirit strives to evolve and assert itself through the actualization of your distinctive inclinations, talents and potentialities. Your life journey is an individual story of ongoing efforts toward spiritual expression and personal transformation.

Spirit is the essential transforming power in our lives. It expresses itself through human joys and sorrows projected in human behavior and different life styles. Spirit is the animating element of life in your heart, mind and body and is the origin of your zest and enthusiasm. A person in good spirits is perceived as healthy and delightful, while a person in poor spirits tends toward depression, apathy and ill health. Many religions have taught that God is the great creative Spirit moving within and around us in wondrous ways and forms.

Create in me a clean heart, O God;
and renew a right spirit within me.
Cast me not away from thy presence;
and take not thy holy spirit from me.
Restore unto me the joy of thy salvation;
and uphold me with thy free spirit.
-Psalm 51: 10-12

Personal happiness and the continued development of civilization depends on the nourishment and healthy expression of the human spirit within each of us. Many poets, such as Shakespeare, have celebrated the quickness and freshness of the spirit of love. As humans, we especially grow and thrive through such deep emotional expressions as love, care, hope, kindness, faith, joy and celebration. Each unique spirit is also projected into the world about us in the creation of cultural communities with highly distinctive forms of art, music, literature, science and technology.

- SPIRITUAL HUMOR -

Does God have a sense of humor? He must have if he made us!
-Jackie Gleason

I enjoy a good laugh - one that rushes out of one's soul like the breaking up of a Sunday school.
-Josh Billings

I believe in laughter, I think it's food for the soul!
-Tommy Lasorda

Only two things are infinite, the universe and human stupidity, and I'm not sure about the former.
-Albert Einstein

God help those who do not help themselves!
-Addison Mizner

Jesus died too soon. He would have repudiated his doctrine if he had lived to my age.
-Friedrich Nietzsche

Humor is the prelude to faith and laughter is the beginning of prayer.
-Reinhold Niebuhr

God cannot be solemn or he would not have blessed humans with the incalculable gift of laughter.
-Sydney Harris

I'm astounded by people who want to "know" the universe when it's hard enough to find your way around Chinatown.
-Woody Allen

Laughter is the celebration of the human spirit.
-Sabina White

My desire for knowledge is intermittent;
but my desire to commune with the spirit of the universe,
to be intoxicated even with the fumes, call it of that divine nectar,
to bear my head through atmospheres and over heights unknown to my feet,
is perennial and constant.
-Henry David Thoreau

But the Spirit of life surrounds us in numerous other forms which also move us with awe and veneration. The boundless beauty and fruits of nature enrich and renew us when we commune with kindred spirits around us. We are all moved and inspired by the grandeur of oceans, majestic mountains, beautiful flowers, birdsong and the companionship of other animals. Indeed, much personal unhappiness can be attributed to ignorance of or antipathy toward nature.

O Great Spirit
Give me strength to walk the soft earth.
Give me the eyes to see and the strength to understand.
-BlackElk

We are all uniquely inspired when we have been infused with a special breath of life which newly arouses and impels us to creative thought and action. Inspiration springs from the depths of soulful reflection and contemplation which excites and impels us to new heights of creative endeavor. When we reflect on the wonders of nature, the beauty of art and music, stimulating literature or the great thoughts of men or women, we are reinvigorated with spiritual energy to meet the demands of our day.

Examples abound. William Shakespeare, in Sonnet 86, referred to his own creative spirit as an "affable familiar ghost which nightly gulls him with intelligence." This spirit lies primarily within the unconscious personality itself and not just in the logical mind - but is eventually displayed in both emotional and rational forms, such as Dante's Divine Comedy and Goethe's Faust. In modern times we are surrounded with the results of artistic and scientific endeavors which are the results of uniquely human creative spirits. It is our spirits and passions which make us live and utilize whatever knowledge and wisdom we may possess at the time to cope with daily tasks and challenges.

The power of the human spirit is continuously demonstrated in numerous ways. Spirit is a form of energy that can be expressed in both positive and negative forms such as creative evolution or destructive acts. We are able to actualize and direct our own spirits through consciously directed thoughts and actions. Thinking positively and imaginatively is the first step to health and wholeness. When we think negatively, we quickly become emotionally and spiritually upset which can result in personal dis-ease, illness and social problems.

Many philosophers and scientists have attempted to explain how some spiritual thoughts or positive "notions in our head" drive us to constructive action. The discoveries of quantum physicists suggest mind and matter are inseparable and that the probability of something happening depends on the way that we think and perceive. It appears that our personal universe and sense of reality may actually be determined by a combination of electro-magnetic waves, gravity, nuclear forces, *conscious choices* - and other forces yet to be discovered.

Quantum physics indicated that between actual observations, the world exists not as a solid actuality but only as shimmering waves of possibility.
-Nick Herbert

We are now aware that many forms of energy, such as atomic elements, contain both positive and negative charges which are continuously changing. For example, a proton is a positively charged physical particle while an electron is negatively charged - both of them balancing each other in relatively stable physical forms of matter. On the other hand, a photon is a quantum of electromagnetic energy that demonstrates both wavelike and particle behavior but has no charge and possesses momentum. Other forms of energy are yet to be understood.

For instance, a *"psitron"* can be posited as the smallest instrument of consciously directed energy in the human psyche (and other life forms) through the direct means of mental or spiritual thoughts. Perhaps some of the effects of positive or negative "psitrons" are already being measured in self-concept scales, colored Kirlian and magnetic brain resonance photographs, etc. However, our never ending spiritual problem is how to expand and control our conscious self-awareness and knowledge of the forces within ourselves and the universe - in order to assure continuation of both personal and social evolution.

The great sea has set me in motion, set me
moving like a weed in a river adrift,
The sky and the strong wind have moved the Spirit inside me
till I am carried away trembling with joy.
-Uvavnuk

Through time immemorial, we have also accumulated the wisdom and insights of inspired men and women who may continue to personally influence us as spiritual guides and models for what we may yet become. Solomon prayed that the spirit of wisdom might come to him and we are still guided by his reflections and insights as recorded in the Bible. Other great spiritual leaders, such as Lao Tzu, Buddha, Moses, Jesus, Mohammed, Emerson, Gandhi and Martin Luther King, Jr., have continued to guide us with their thoughts, prayers and lives. Sometimes we are also inspired by the spirit and determination of certain family members, friends, acquaintances and personal heroes of all kinds who have helped to show us another way to a better life.

I love love - though he has wings
and like light can flee.
But above all other things,
Spirit, I love thee!
-Percy Bysshe Shelley

Humans are also inspired by mythical heroes who appear in the stories and great literature of their civilization. All cultures have their own creation stories and subsequent prophets to guide them through the life journey. Myths, dreams, fairy tales and modern science fiction continue to portray the unusual powers inherent in projections of the human spirit in certain times and places. Most of these stories record how the hero successfully overcame great hardship through spiritual fortitude, courage, determination, hope and faith in special help from gods.

Be ye lamps unto yourselves.
Be your own confidence.
Hold to the truth within yourselves
as to the only lamp.
-Buddha

For example, hope is the feeling that what is needed or strongly desired will someday be realized - or at least that life will get better with continued work and perseverance. One of the great myths of all time emphasized the importance of hope in our lives. Jupiter is the king of the ancient Greek gods who bestowed many gifts on humankind. In order to help us cope with our many trials and tribulations, Jupiter sent the first woman, Pandora, to give humans a box full of very special spiritual powers. Unfortunately, Pandora opened the box incautiously and, one by one, the spiritual blessings escaped by flying away - but HOPE remained. So, thankfully, even in the most adverse circumstances, hope still springs eternal within the human breast.

Hope is like a rainbow on a very stormy day,
it can help renew us and keep the clouds away.
Hope can also be a dream to which we each aspire
with great expectations that set the spirit afire.
Hope may be a wishing star or such a guiding light
it can point the way to go on a very lonely night.
Hope can be the human key for those who would survive
all trials and tribulations and miraculously still thrive!

There is a Great Spirit within the human soul that enlivens us with a multitude of re-creative inclinations. The human journey consists of daily encounters between the spirits of love and hate, faith and skepticism, hope and despair and myriad others. But we are saved by the spirits of faith, hope and charity which move us to distinctively human actions. It is these positive qualities within the human psyche that enable us to renew and recreate ourselves from day to day and to build a better tomorrow.

I can pass from the happiness of knowledge and virtue
to the eternal calm and joy and peace of the Spirit
when I become one with the highest Self
and with all beings.
-Bhagavad-Gita

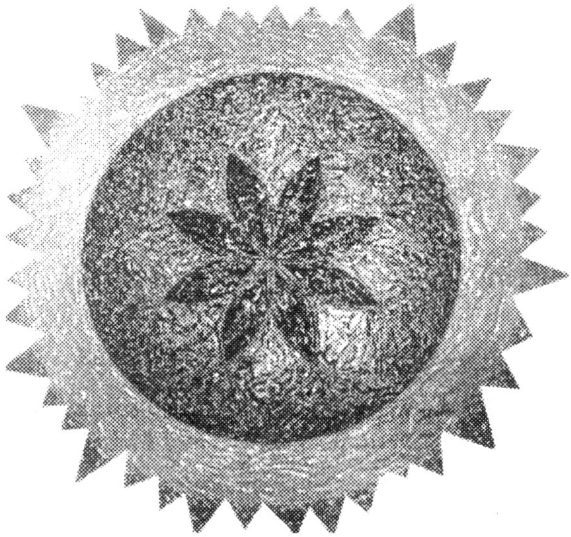

+ MY SPIRIT RISES +

Surrounded by nature's beauty
often I sit for hours,
while my senses feast upon the spectacles of nature.
Here the majestic sun is not concealed
...here the blue sky is my sublime roof.
When in the evening I contemplate the sky in wonder
and the host of luminous bodies
continually revolving within their orbits,
suns or earths by name,
then my spirit rises beyond these constellations
so many millions of miles away.
-Ludwig van Beethoven

A Personal Survey

This is the time to stop and reflect on your own life and spirit by completing the following sentences as rapidly as you can. Express the first thought or feeling that comes to your mind. Make additional comments as needed.

1. My spiritual development really began-
2. I am often inspired by-
3. I continue to hope for-
4. A major passion in my life has been-
5. One of my spiritual guides has been-
6. Some of my spiritual thoughts-
7. I have sometimes been spiritually moved by-
8. The highlights of my human journey have included-
9. The great creative spirit-
10. I believe-

3

---- MIND ----

Seek ye first the good things of the mind, and the rest will either be supplied or its loss will not be felt.
-Francis Bacon

Mind is a *holistic spiritual* agent which integrates and coordinates multitudes of sensory impressions and data emanating from the immediate environment and within the human psyche. The individual human mind operates as a personal psychological system of meaningful adaptation to our unique world of acquired sensory information and knowledge. With conscious effort, focus and attention, associations are made with previously stored impressions, memories and predispositions which finally result in some degree of personal wisdom and *understanding* necessary to adjust to life demands.

Homo sapiens has survived and prospered through the ages because the human mind has been able to quickly comprehend and creatively adjust to the complexities of environmental demands. Over time, the mind develops and establishes significant relationships between sensory patterns, intuitive images, facts and other bits of information. In every person's mind these impressions slowly become organized as words, thoughts, opinions and beliefs which subsequently have directive influence on behavior.

Man is a creature volatile of expression,
and across his features in a day may flow
happiness and remorse, rage and charity.
A flower might open a person's mind-
only man's own mind, especially the artist's mind,
can change the winter in man.
-Loren Eisely

Mind affects the body in several ways. It is the psychic force which integrates and interprets information and makes fundamental choices and decisions based on self-interest and survival. Concomitantly, it proceeds to formulate thoughtful ideals, self-images, goals, purposes, beliefs and aspirations for living and becoming a whole and healthy person. Thoughtful convictions are further confirmed through conscious willful expressions such as affirmations, oaths or other intentional statements or actions.

I want to light up my own mind.
-Robert Browning

What the mind thinks, accepts, and believes moves our *will* to effect specific behavioral actions. The "will to live" in certain ways is then expressed through both conscious and unconscious processes. Conscious willful determination to write a letter, eat, pray, exercise, sing or help another person usually results in some appropriate bodily response. The mindful *will* also operates unconsciously through emotional states where our feelings affect internal bodily functions such as breathing, heart rate, digestion and the immune system. A wise person understands that peace and good health result from the harmonious balance of body, mind and spirit.

Wisdom's self oft seeks to sweet retired solitude, where with her best nurse, Contemplation, she plums her feathers and lets grow her wings.
-John Milton

True wisdom consists of the comprehension, understanding and appropriate use of acquired knowledge and information, which enables us to survive and thrive as the human species. This accumulated wisdom has been recorded in poetry and great literature down through the ages. Proverbial wisdom advises us that, if we think ahead and apply our hearts to instruction and self-knowledge, we will always have hope for the future and be happy. Great leaders and educators, such as President Theodore Roosevelt, have taught that all the resources we need are in the mind!

Happy is the man who finds wisdom
and the man who gets understanding,
for the gain from it is better than gain from silver
and its profit better than gold.
She is more precious than jewels,
and nothing can compare with her.
Long life is in her right hand;
in her left hand are riches and honor.
Her ways are ways of pleasantness
and all her paths are peace.
She is a tree of life to those who lay hold of her;
those who hold her fast are called happy.
-Proverbs 3: 13-18

Let knowledge grow from more to more,
but more of reverence in us dwell;
that mind and soul, according well,
may make one music as before
-Alfred, Lord Tennyson

The human mind has proven to be very suggestible and is subject to both intrinsic self-determination as well as influence and direction from other persons and sources. When we are involved in serious emotional states such as love, fear, strong peer pressures or accidents, our minds may be overwhelmed with instinctual responses. We may also be subject to altered states of mind and consciousness by environmental toxins, substance abuse, music, light and the overwhelming beauty of nature.

Many suggestions and ideas of friends or admired personalities are also absorbed by our unconscious minds. Considerable evidence also supports the power of directive prayer, meditation and positive affirmations on the human mind and body. Scientific studies now confirm the validity of Buddha's words that *all that we are is the result of what we think and believe*. Similarly, the poet Virgil asserted that *mind moves matter*! Because the human mind is distinguished by its tendency for continual growth and evolution of uniquely creative potentialities, it has been attributed with a divine essence.

Philosophers have asserted that true "mind" is formed when the individual demonstrates some capability of creating images, "trains of thought" or ideas. The highest effort or function of the mind is to understand the fundamental nature of things through the acquisition or growth of personal knowledge and to continually transform this information into newly creative forms and endeavors.

I have felt a presence that disturbs me with the joy of elevated thoughts;
a sense sublime of something far more deeply interfused,
whose dwelling is the light of setting suns,
and the round ocean and the living air,
and the blue sky, and in the mind of man.
-William Wordsworth

Civilization itself is the product of uniquely creative human minds and endeavors. That the human mind contains mysterious powers yet to be developed and better understood is evidenced through the recorded experience of such great personalities as Jesus, Swedenborg, William Wordsworth, Abraham Lincoln, Mark Twain and countless others.

I am forced to believe that one human mind can communicate with another, over any sort of distance without any artificial conditions acting as a transmitting agent. Doubtless the something which conveys our thoughts through the air from brain to brain is a finer and subtler form of electricity, and all we need to do is to find how to capture it and how to force it to do its work.

-Mark Twain

Through cultural experience the human mind emerges as distinctive notions, images, dreams, visions, concepts and ideas commonly expressed through art, literature, music, science and technology. The modern human mind contains amazingly positive and creative proclivities for personal growth, construction, healing and renewal. But it also contains many dark unconscious evolutionary potentialities which, when expressed in deliberately evil tendencies to injure, kill and destroy, creates havoc with our rational world order and civilized presumptions.

Your mind is a psychic structure similar to an archeological mound; upon investigation, the upper easily accessible layer of artifacts and remnants of recent times is analogous to your conscious state of awareness. The deeper subterranean archeological layers contain broken and fused materials comparable to the instinctual biological tendencies of the evolutionary mind buried in the collective human unconscious. Similarly, Sigmund Freud portrayed the mind as an iceberg floating with only one-seventh of its bulk above the water in the conscious light of day, while most of its forceful mass is submerged in the dark ocean.

The growth of the mind and human consciousness is a never ending evolutionary process of molecular genetics, cultural development and education. As illustrated on the opposite page, this process can be visualized as an ancient sequoia or giant cedar tree which has gradually emerged from the global unconscious powers inherent in the earthy seeds of nature. Eventually, distinctive human beings and their cultures are formed and forever leave their imprint on our collective unconscious. But in due time, natural inclinations are shaped through experience and deliberate training. Finally, individual personal consciousness appears and expands interdependently with specific enviromental factors and cosmic forces.

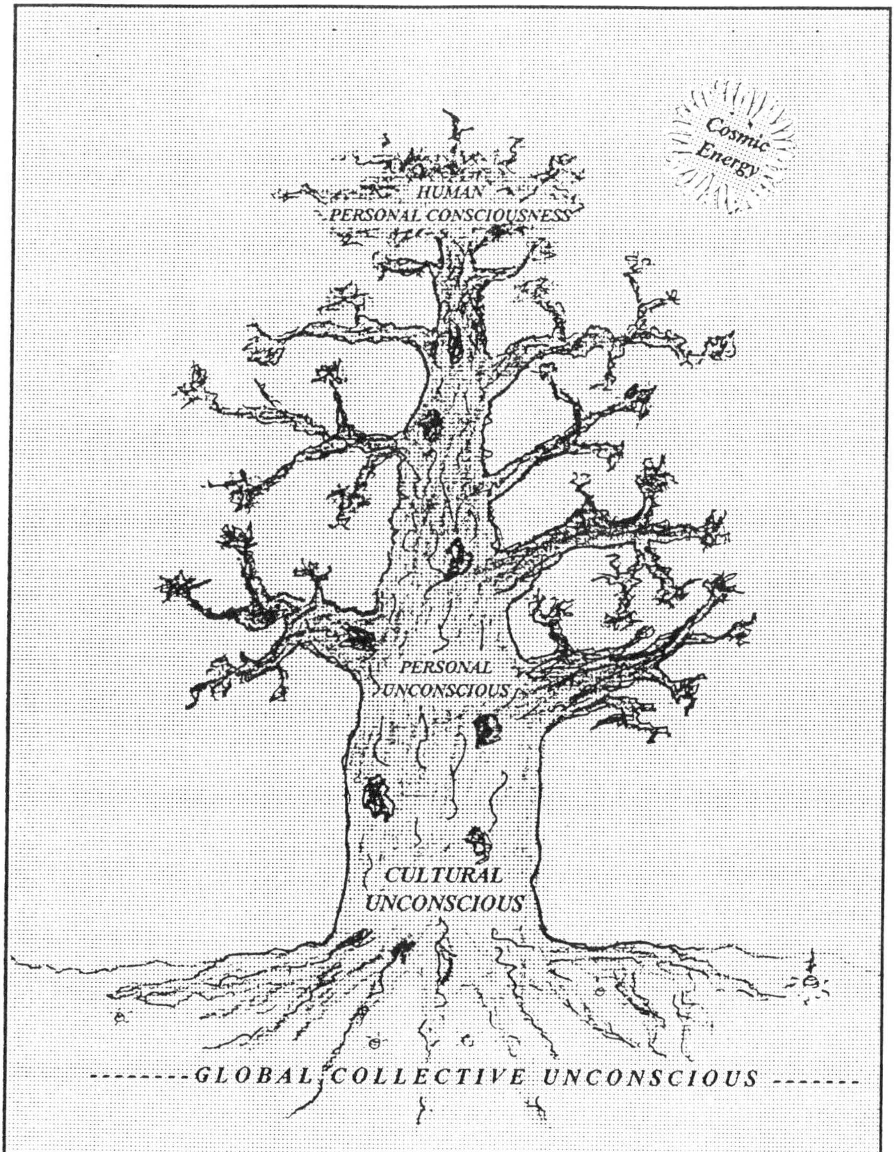

THE GROWTH OF MIND AND HUMAN CONSCIOUSNESS

Poetry was ever thought to have some participation in divineness, because it doth raise and erect the mind.
-Francis Bacon

Amazingly, most of the time the brain works in harmony with the body in a holistic processing and meaningful integration of complex sensory data from numerous energy spectrums such as light, pressure, sound, smell, taste, gravity and others not yet clearly understood. In fact, both our immaterial thoughts and the physical organs of our bodies are comprised of rapidly interacting electromagnetic and chemical forces that are forever changing and renewing. Sometimes, unfortunately, this harmonious interaction is disrupted by illness and disease which may impair one's state of mind and being.

The mind does affect the body through deliberate conscious acts of willful design and effort, but it also operates unconsciously through our physiological intelligence and emotional states. A major challenge in life should be how to light up, constantly renew and expand one's own mind. If we have sound minds in sound bodies we tend to be healthy, positive and blossoming. We always have latent potentialities and powers yet to be developed such as unique talents, special forms of creative expression, constructive visions, precognition, telepathy, cosmic consciousness, predispositions and other states of enlightenment.

Through eons of time, nature has provided mankind with creatively aspiring minds and inclinations. We are wiser than we consciously know or understand. As unique living creatures, we continuously contemplate our origins and undertake to design the future through the assertion of will and effort. Many religious persons also believe that the human mind is forever striving to express its manifold potentialities as a special gift of God and its end is to become reunited with the universal Mind or cosmic Soul. Although some of these philosophical ideas may be unverifiable to subjectively limited human perception and knowledge, they will forever remain as mysteriously compelling speculations and psychic forces throughout our lives.

We should keep in mind that our personal visible world is just a part of a broader universe from which it draws its chief significance - harmonious relations and final union with that higher universe is our true end.
-William James

+++ WILL +++

There is no chance, no destiny, no fate,
Can circumvent or hinder or control
The firm resolve of a determined soul.

Gifts count for nothing; will alone is great;
All things give way before it, soon or late.

What obstacle can stay the mighty force
Of the sea-seeking river in its course,
Or cause the ascending orb of day to wait?

Each well-born soul must win what it deserves.
Let the fool prate of luck.

The fortunate is he whose earnest purpose never swerves,
Whose slightest action or inaction serves
The one great aim.
Why, even death stands still,
And waits an hour sometimes
For such a will.
-Ella Wheeler Wilcox

A Personal Survey

This is the time to stop and reflect on your own life and mind by completing the following sentences as rapidly as you can. Express the first thought or feeling that comes to your mind. Make additional comments as needed.

1. Sometimes I feel that my mind-

2. A great influence on my mental development has been-

3. I can always help to "light up" my own mind by-

4. One of my outstanding teachers taught me-

5. At times my unconscious mind-

6. Great books-

7. What I would really like to know is-

8. What helps focus my attention is-

9. I believe I can continue to expand my mind by-

10. To me "true wisdom" means-

4

-----BODY----

Dust thou art, and unto dust shalt thou return. -Genesis 3:19

The human body has developed over 5 billion years of evolution of life on the planet earth. This evolution has resulted from the constant bombardment of trillions of cosmic rays emanating from the sun and the residue of exploding stars. We have, in fact, evolved from the interaction of actual stardust with other natural forces in our unique earthly environment.

Over eons of time, electrons, protons, neutrinos, photons and other mysterious atomic forces have slowly formed, shaped and constantly changed the human body into a sensing and thinking organism capable of affecting its own destiny. The human genus, Homo, is only about 2 million years old while our species, Homo sapiens, is even a more recent evolutionary arrival that is between 100,000 and 200,000 years old.

During this time, the individual human lifespan of about half a century or so has been relatively short but fruitful! *As for man, his days are as grass: as a flower of the field, so he flourisheth* (Psalm 103:15). In his short time on this planet, man has successfully adapted because of the development of a significantly larger brain than other primates. But it is our distinctive forebrain which has enabled us to plan ahead and creatively transform ourselves and the world in which we live.

What a piece of work is a man!
how noble in reason!
how infinite in faculty!
in form and moving how express and admirable!
in action how like an angel!
in apprehension how like a god!
the beauty of the world! the paragon of animals!
-Shakespeare (Hamlet)

But the brain itself remains an imperfect instrument with different levels of perceptual operation and creative thinking -including primitive emotional animalistic instincts toward irrationality. There is also much more to our world and the universe than what we can perceive through our brains and sensory organs. For instance, we directly sense only a small part of the broad electromagnetic spectrum and recognize that many other animals (dogs, bats, birds) respond to frequencies of energy to which we are incapable of responding.

Throughout numerous galaxies in cosmic space, other advanced life forms may also exist and be subject to similar limitations of time and place. Amazingly, with all of our physical limitations, we have developed mental capabilities which help us to better understand our origins and to be able to mold the future in accordance with our dreams of things that might yet be.

All that is of the body is as coursing waters, all that is of the soul as dreams and vapours; life is a warfare, a brief soujourning in an alien land. Where then can man find the power to guide and guard his steps? In one thing and alone: the love of knowledge.
-Marcus Aurelius

However, we have gradually learned that the entire human body, including the brain, is a holistic organism of which the very form and operation is largely determined by genetic endowment and molecular biology. Trillions of cells go to make up the human body. Millions of cells die every minute while millions more are being born, grow and change. The nucleus of each cell contains a complex of molecular building blocks comprised of protein and DNA (deoxyribonucleic acid) which form all 23 pairs of human chromosomes.

The instructions for making a human being comprise some 4 billion nucleotide pairs which produce highly unique hereditary traits in each person. Over periods of time, our genetic structure is gradually changed as a result of natural adaptation, bisexual reproduction, cosmic mutations, infection and other forces yet to be clearly understood. Throughout your life, your unique genetic makeup continues to affect your heart, mind, body and soul in mystifying ways.

The secret sympathy,
the silver link, the silken tie,
which heart to heart, and mind to mind,
in body and in soul can bind.
-Sir Walter Scott

The brain is the main physiological organ for neuropsychological processing of sensory information in the body. We have discovered that certain mental operations and functions are processed in specific parts of the brain. For example, stimulated neurons in the right temporal lobe give rise to visions of light. The left cerebral hemisphere dominates in most logical and rational tasks such as reading and calculating. The right hemisphere is more specialized in non-linear sensory processing such as art and music. The forebrain is concerned with thoughtful planning, the ability to pursue future ends and the choice of their attainment. But the physical brain itself must not be confused with the immaterial human "mind" which is the holistic organizing "*spirit of understanding*" involving the entire body.

"Mind" then depends upon a healthy brain to properly associate sensory data to produce adaptive associations and sequences of ideas. The actual physical "mind-stuff" consists largely of molecular biochemical interactions which occur when sensory information is processed neuropsychologically - which then results in some form of mental awareness and thoughtful behavior. The mind and body also cooperate to combat illness through the immune system which produces special cells that can destroy infecting agents. Included within the immune system are the brain, the spleen, the thymus gland, bone marrow and the lymph nodes. As a whole, the immune system is largely a force-field sensitive to stress-related biochemicals mediated through the hypothalamus and adrenal glands.

The immune system is influenced by strong emotions and by biochemical changes in the body as a result of infection, toxicity and diet. Many biochemicals manufactured in the brain, such as neuropeptides and others, are subject to the person's state-of-mind. Scientific research has now established that strong positive emotions, such as hope, love, will to live, purpose and playfulness, are all powerful psychological forces which affect brain-body chemistry. These thoughts and emotions also directly affect the functioning of the heart and other vital organs.

The heart and the blood circulation system are the major parts of the body's internal transportation system. As an electrically-activated pump, the heart contracts rhythmically to impel the blood through thousands of miles of arteries, microscopic capillaries and veins. Beating about 70 times a minute in resting individuals, the heart propels oxygenated blood from the lungs to all parts of the body where cells are constantly being rejuvenated with vital energy. Throughout this process, the healthy operation of the heart depends on such things as genetic predisposition, diet, physical stress and numerous emotional and psychological factors. Personal beliefs, attitudes and habits, such as exercise, nutrition, smoking , meditation and life style, all affect the heart in one way or another.

-A BIRTHDAY-

My heart is like a singing bird
Whose nest is in a watered shoot;
My heart is like an apple-tree
Whose boughs are bent with thickest fruit;
My heart is like a rainbow shell
That paddles in a halcyon sea;
My heart is gladder than all these
Because my love is come to me.

-Christina G. Rossetti

Psychophysiologically, the words of our mouths and the meditations of our hearts reflect the human spirit of life. The wisdom of the human heart actually feels things the eyes cannot see and knows what the mind cannot understand. This has long been recognized and celebrated by the poets and musicians of every age. We respond to personal loss or tragedy with heart aches which can become very life threatening. And the heart leaps with joy when we feel the beauty of love or nature. Great poets and musicians have noted that the heart, body and soul are intertwined in life and death.

The entire body is forever adapting to the demands of time, place, thoughts and action. Symbolic thought and language are the major products of brain functioning which propels the body to action. But there is a special wisdom inherent in other parts of the body, such as the immune system, the heart, the digestive organs and cellular functions, which also move us to feel and act appropriately.

How good is man's life, the mere living!
how fit to employ all the heart
and the soul and the senses,
forever in joy!
-Robert Browning

Biblically, the entire human body has been described as the physical temple of the "Holy Ghost" within us - since the outward manifestations of the body tend to reflect the holistic life spirit in all of its parts. Carl Jung, a great psychologist, also professed that the body is but the outward manifestation of this vital spirit within us.

Amazingly, most of the time our body organs work cooperatively while processing complex sensory information data and executing appropriate responses. There is little doubt but that a healthy state of being is truly the result of an energizing harmony between one's mind, body and spirit.

-I Sing The Body Electric -

Was it doubted that those who corrupt their own bodies
conceal themselves?
And if the body does not do as much as the Soul?
And if the body were not Soul, what is the Soul?

If anything is sacred, the human body is sacred...
O my Body! I believe the likes of you are to stand
or fall with the likes of the Soul...
Head...eyes...mouth...nose...strong shoulders...ribs...
The lungs-sponges...the stomach sac...the brain in its folds
inside the skull-frame...
The exquisite realization of health;

O I say, these are not the parts and poems of the Body only,
but of the Soul.
- Walt Whitman

-A Personal Survey-

This is the time to stop and reflect on your own life and body by completing the following sentences as rapidly as you can. Express the first thought or feeling that comes to your mind. Make additional comments as needed.

1. My general physical characteristics are -
2. One of my physical assets is -
3. My most serious limitation is -
4. Sometimes my heart -
5. I anticipate my personal longevity to be -
6. Some of my genetic predispositions seem to be -
7. My resistance to disease depends on -
8. I am really propelled to action when -
9. Sometimes I feel my spirit affects my body when -
10. My physical evolution -

5

----SOUL----

For what has a man profited, if he shall gain the whole world, and lose his own soul?
- Matthew 16:26

The soul has been commonly defined as the divine spark which invigorates human life. It is of immortal cosmic origins, containing both positive and negative powers inherent in creative acts and moral inclinations. Your soul is a unique seed-like dynamic spiritual force which guides your human morphogenetic qualities into bodily form, structure, thought and action. As such, it is the seat of your deepest emotions, unconscious predispositions, knowledge and insights.

Being that has soul is a *living* being. Soul is the essential vital force in humankind which lives of itself and causes life. As the universal animating vital force in life, the soul is an immaterial ghost in the human machine. However, the soul may be more accurately conceived as the dynamic but silent unconscious spectator behind every human choice and act which effects the body, mind and spirit.

Many persons subscribe to the views of the early philosopher-physician, Paracelus, who stated that the vital soul is not enclosed in persons, but radiates about and through us over time and events and may produce healthy or morbid effects according to our thoughts and imaginations. In this sense, the "Soul" is part of the great spaceless, universal cosmic force or creative "God" within all things.

- THE OVERSOUL -

There is a deep power in which we exist and whose beautitude is accessible to us. It comes to whoever will put off what is foreign and proud; it comes as serenity and grandeur.
Within us is the soul of the whole; the wise silence, the universal beauty to which every part and particle is equally related; the eternal One.
When it breaks through our intellect, it is genius;
when it breathes through our will, it is virtue;
when it flows through our affections, it is love.
-Ralph Waldo Emerson

Some modern neuroscientists have agreed that many attempts to understand human behavior are incomplete failures of imagination if they fail to take into account the spiritual element in life. Research into the workings of the human nervous system eventually leads to an *energizing* forceful soul. This vital force also appears to vary according to life stages and circumstances.

Robertson Davies, a renowned novelist, describes the human journey as a Pilgrim's Progress through developmental stages. The individual soul moves through life beginning with infantile fantasies and adolescent preoccupation with the physical concerns of youth. Then, in adulthood, it begins to encounter logical principles, metaphysics and skepticism.

As a result of ongoing human struggles and dilemmas, by the time most of us reach middle age our human journey results in accumulated wisdom and maturity. This process of gradually becoming a more completely balanced and realized person is the culmination of the soul's quest for evolution and wholeness in this life.

I Believe In You My Soul.
The Soul travels; the body does not travel as much as the soul;
the body has just as great a work as the Soul
- and parts away for the progress of Souls;
all that was or is apparent upon this globe or any globe,
fall into niches and corners before the procession of souls
along the grand roads of the universe.
-Walt Whitman

Finally, through the use of creative imagination the person achieves some degree of psychological balance and a unified view of life, resulting from the synthesis of unconscious fantasy, scientific knowledge and moral mythology. This gradually acquired wisdom then meets in a religious reconciliation of the soul with the realistic demands of daily life.

Our birth is but a sleep and a forgetting-
the soul that rises with us; our life's star
hath elsewhere its setting.
- William Wordsworth

As part of the universal Over-Soul we are subject to its laws of creation, growth and change. But humankind is unique in its self-consciousness and ability to communicate through language and creative endeavors. As a result, we can consciously participate in how and where we invest our life energies which help determine what we become. Through our personal choices and resulting actions, we also have an impact on evolutionary trends and the course of civilization itself.

I believe that man will not merely endure: he will prevail.
He is immortal, not because he alone among creatures
has an inexhaustible voice, but because he has a soul,
a spirit capable of compassion and sacrifice and endurance.
-William Faulkner

Chinese philosophers long ago recognized the importance of primal creative forces operating in nature and humankind. They called the positive active element Yang and the negative passive element Yin; the interaction of these two forces is said to produce all life and change. Vital life energy is attributed to the flow of these forces through the body, with a proper balance of positive and negative elements resulting in harmony and good health. The flow of universal forces from the great soul within you can be somewhat controlled by personal practices, such as directed breathing, meditation and special physical and mental exercises.

-TAO-
Before the Heaven and the Earth existed there was something nebulous:
Silent, isolated, standing alone,
changing not, eternally revolving without fail,
worthy to be the Mother of all things.
I do not know its name and address it as Tao.
If forced to give it a name,
I shall call it "Great"
The Great Tao flows everywhere.
-Lao Tzu

I am the soul of nature that gives life to the universe.
From Me all things proceed and unto me they must return.
And you who seek to know me,
know that your seeking and yearning will avail you not,
unless you know the mystery:
for if that which you seek,
you find not within yourself,
you will never find it without.
-Starhawk

Modern psychology has also helped us understand the nature of productive psychic energy uniquely expressed through our hopes, dreams, art, work and continual creative endeavors. William James was one of the first great psychologists who concluded that our own personal thoughts and affirmations are forces which are responded to by universal powers flowing through us.

How we pray, think and act can enrich our souls and improve the lives of others. Hippocrates taught that feeding the soul is as important as feeding the body. Since the human Soul is the basic source of personal spirit, zest and enthusiasm which distinguishes individuality, it must be nurtured and renewed from time to time with care and attention. With contemplated effort a wholesome life can result from the soulful integration of one's body, mind and spirit.

*****

The Lord is my shepherd; I shall not want.
He maketh me to lie down in green pastures:
he leadeth me beside the still water.
He restoreth my Soul:
He leadeth me in the paths of righteousness for his names sake.
Yea, though I walk through the valley of the shadow of death,
I will fear no evil: for thou art with me.
Thou preparest a table before me in the presence of mine enemies:
thou anointest my head with oil;
my cup runneth over.
Surely goodness and mercy shall follow me all the days of my life;
and I will dwell in the house of the Lord for ever.
-Psalm 23

+++ THE SOUL +++

All are but parts of one stupendous whole,
whose body nature is, and God the soul.
-Alexander Pope

The body's mischiefs as Plato proves, proceed from the soul:
and if the mind be not first satisfied, the body can never be cured.
-Anon

Character cannot be developed in ease and quiet.
Only through experiences of trial and suffering
can the soul be strengthened, vision cleared,
ambition inspired and success achieved.
-Helen Keller

Confessions may be good for the soul
but they are bad for the reputation.
-Thomas R. Dewar

The principal thing in this world is to keep one's soul aloft.
-Gustave Flaubert

How good is man's life, the mere living!
how fit to employ all the heart and the soul and the senses,
for ever in joy!
-Elizabeth Barrett Browning

I am that which began; out of me the years roll;
out of me God and man; I am equal and whole;
God changes and man, and the form of them bodily;
I am the soul.
-Algernon Charles Swinburne

All science is a function of the soul,
in which all knowledge is rooted.
-Carl G. Jung

+++ SOUL POWER +++

Purpose: To explore personal dimensions of your soul.

Procedure: Concentrate on these words as you sit or lie in a relaxed position or tape record your own voice for more reflective listening.

Let yourself be quiet and relaxed. Begin to breathe slowly and deeply as your entire body gradually becomes more calm and restful. Feel any tension draining from your body as you become more serene. Now focus your mental energy on the inner center of your very being . Imagine yourself sitting in a quiet and beautiful spot outdoors under the broad and expansive starlit sky. Feel wonderfully at ease throughout your entire body.

You are alone but feeling mellow and at ease as you gaze at the awesome sight of the majestic blue starlit sky surrounding you. Now envision your soul as a divine spark of life within you, glistening with unique creative potentialities. Imagine your soul as beautiful pulsating starlight, emanating powerful spiritual forces of vitality throughout your mind and body. Feel this soulpower stirring your entire being to realize its unique potentialities throughout the universe.

Visualize your vital soul power reaching out to the universe around and above you. Your soul is glowing and lighting the way as it slowly ascends through space and time. Within your entire being, you feel in the process of transformation, of becoming an even more vital part of the awesome universe about you. Now imagine your unique soul as being infused with regenerating cosmic forces. Slowly become aware of the interchange of transcending creative energy between you and the mysterious totality of which you are a part. You are glowing with potentiality!

In your mind's eye envision yourself harmoniously merging with the vast cosmos surrounding you. Now see your vibrant soul metamorphosing and continually changing into untold possibilities. Feel yourself as a great creative part of the evolving universe. You are a special human changeling endowed with mighty godlike forces within you that are transforming your spirit and joy of life.

Now quietly repeat your name and feel uniquely in touch with your entire body, mind and soul. Imagine that your creative spirit is rejuvenated and empowered. Gradually let yourself come back to present time and space and feel grateful for the soulpower that enables you to celebrate the joy of life!

A Personal Survey

This is the time to stop and reflect on your own life and soul by completing the following sentences as rapidly as you can. Express the first thought or feeling that comes to your mind. Make additional comments as needed.

1. My soul-

2. I have attempted to "feed and enrich" my soul by-

3. Some music that stirs my soul is-

4. A unique thing about my soul is-

5. At times I try to commune with my soul by-

6. Real "soul food" to me includes-

7. I most often express my soul through-

8. My mind, body and soul-

9. Some great souls-

10. I believe that my soul-

6

----- LOVING CARE -----

You shall love your neighbor as yourself.
- Leviticus 19:17

Love is a deep and tender feeling of attachment, care and devotion. It has instinctual roots in our biological drive to reproduce, the nurturance of our offspring and the mutual care we provide one another in order to survive and flourish. True love is the result of strong emotional attraction that grows from common concerns, interests, values, physical care and bonding over time and experience. Mature love gradually develops as a result of continued care, understanding, acceptance and commitment. When loving care is mutually provided and nourished over good times and bad, real companionship is strengthened.

Love one another, but make not a bond of love;
Let it be a moving sea between the shores of your souls.
- Kahlil Gibran

Jesus and other great religious leaders taught that love is the most powerful spiritual force in the world. As a spiritual force, human love is uniquely experienced and passionately felt throughout one's entire being. But the essence of true love is centered in the psychological relationship of bonded souls and is intensely felt in their hearts, minds and bodies.

Without love, our lives lack deep personal interdependency and connection, from which we derive essential joy, meaning and purpose. Biblical wisdom states that, without love, we are nothing but hollow vessels. Our life's journey is a continual quest for love and fulfillment.

Love is patient; love is kind and envies no one.
Love is never boastful nor conceited, nor rude;
never selfish, not quick to take offense.
Love keeps no score of wrongs;
does not gloat over other men's sins, but delights in the truth.
There is nothing love cannot face;
there is no limit to its faith, its hope, and its endurance.
- 1 Corinthians 13:4-7

The trouble with a lot of marriages is that the husband is so busy bringing home the bacon that he forgets the applesauce.
- Dan Bennett

True love is never easy, nor does it always bring joy and happiness. The many heartaches and disappointments of love must be recognized. These include rejection or unrequited affection, jealousy and favoritism. The intense feelings of hate, revenge and spite are visible realities of the opposites of true love and we risk these when we expose ourselves intimately to others.

Fortunately, we can always learn from the mistakes of frustrated love and, sometimes, another marriage is the triumph of hope and acquired wisdom over a bad experience. With all of the difficulties involved, loving shared relationships are more productive of happiness. Married men and women consistently report being happier than people who are single, divorced or widowed and they also tend to live longer and healthier lives.

But love is such a mystery,
I cannot find it out:
For when I think I'm best resolv'd,
I then am most in doubt.
Once upon it, I have loved
three whole days together;
and am like to love three more,
if it prove fair weather.
- John Suckling

As Shakespeare noted, at least initially, love tends to be blind and lovers cannot seem to see the petty follies that they themselves commit. But true love only flowers from deliberate cultivation and prolonged nurturance. The feelings of mutually loving hearts and minds, unlike infatuation or mere lust, remain long after the temporary heat of passion has gone. And with the sharing of joys and sorrows, loving companions gradually learn to accept their mutual faults, deficiencies and limitations. Then, as soulmates, they accept and enable each other to become more complete and balanced persons.

Let us strive more to comfort others than to be comforted,
to understand others, than to be understood,
to love others more than to be loved.
For it is in giving that we receive,
and in forgiving that we are forgiven.
- St. Francis of Assisi

With proper care, we gradually learn to love and be loved. A mother's love for her children, infant love and dependence on the mother and adult sexual love and attachment are all basic representations of this life force. So too is fatherly love commonly expressed in concern and protection of the family and cultural group. Other forms include the love of and attachment to friends which help us to multiply our joys and share our sorrows. We also experience many kinds of love - of country, of life, of nature and of God.

Our never ending need for love helps us reach out to our fellow beings and contributes to the building of the larger caring human community. The spirit of love extends from progressive attachments to self, family, community and, finally, to the natural universe itself. What is important is that we open ourselves to the creative powers of this great spiritual force and learn to love as fully as we can.

Praise be the fathomless universe, for life and joy,
and for objects and knowledge curious.
and for love, sweet love.
- Walt Whitman

Our inner spirit of life is renewed daily by faith, hope, admiration and love. Whatever the risk of intimate personal involvement, it is essential that we deliberately cultivate our unique potentiality for loving *care* of self and others. The foundation of human love is intimate care which is expressed in positive regard, concern, and nurturance. However, in order to be able to truly love others we must first be able to love ourselves - as evidenced by self-respect, care, and the furtherance of our own human potentialities. Only then are we psychologically able to reach out and try to love our neighbors as ourselves.

+ Psalm To My Beloved +
Lo, I have opened unto you the wide gates of my being,
And like a tide you have flowed into me.
The innermost recesses of my spirit are full of you,
and all the channels of my soul are
grown sweet with your presence.
- Eunice Tietjens

Many cultures have promulgated the basic ethical admonition to love your neighbor as yourself. This presupposes that most persons do care for, promote and nurture themselves and feel that it is desirable to extend this behavior toward others. Many parents, for instance, hopefully strive to care for their children in the way they would like to have been cared for when they were children. When such positive care, respect and regard is held for self and then extended to others, love becomes a transforming force in human life.

Self-love is expressed by acts of attention, care and nurturance that we give to ourselves. The way you treat your body and cultivate your mind and soul is a reflection of self esteem. Personal hygiene, nutrition, sleep and relaxation, educational endeavors and leisure time pursuits are all indicators of just how well you love and care for your Self.

When you provide proper attention to your Self, you find it to be enjoyable and satisfying. The things we most enjoy can be used as self-incentives for continued personal development. When you effectively love yourself you can then both give and receive love from others.

Self-Love but serves the virtuous Mind to wake,
as the small pebble stirs the peaceful lake;
the center moved, a circle strait succeeds,
another still, and still another spreads,
friend, parent, neighbor, first it will embrace,
his county next, and next all human race;
Wide and morewide, the overflowing of the Mind
takes every creature in of everykind.
- Anon

Learning to love more fully demands considerable time and effort in coming to know, understand and care for one's own needs before being able to reach out and establish intimate contact with another person. True self-love and respect are thereby reflected in the care and comfort we give to significant other persons and the wider community in which we live. When we love, care for and help others to develop or realize their own human potentialities, we are rewarded with joyful feelings of personal transcendence and goodness.

Love is truly a magical something that, when we give it away, we wind up having more. Reinhold Niebuhr elucidates this by explaining that nothing that we do, however virtuous, is accomplished alone and therefore we are spiritually saved by acts of love. When we are good to others, we are also best to ourselves; when we sincerely try to help and care for others, we become more fully balanced and realized human beings.

A loving and balanced person is also in harmony with nature and the universe itself. When we are true to ourselves, we feel fully alive and at one with the flow of life in and about us. As guardian stewards of this beautiful earth and its wonderfully diverse forms of life, we can extend our loving care and protection to other creatures of the earth and to the planet itself. Thus do we nourish and contribute to the betterment of human life itself. Our personal actions help determine the future and the fruitfulness of the world of which we are a part.

We interdependently nurture children, other persons, growing things and the global environment. The streams, trees, fields and flowers teem with life and fruits that help nourish and sustain us. As we love and care for these natural elements, we affect our own joy and quality of life. Through caring conservation of life and nature, we become more in harmony with the total universe. The loving care of nature also brings us immediate reciprocal rewards and special feelings of earthly peace and contentment.

I come and go with a strange liberty in nature. There can be no very black melancholy to him who lives in the midst of nature.

- Henry David Thoreau

Oh God, I thank you for buttered slices of sunlight
and the toasted air warming me.
- Rececca Roberts

Sometimes we are awed by the glory of beautiful sunsets or other unusual experiences which help us to realize the joy and miracle of being alive and able to care deeply about such things. This special love of God's creation, and the wonderful mysteries of nature, can renew our spirits through a sense of cosmic harmony and personal transcendence. We are an integral part of the natural universe inseparably intertwined with all life forms on this spaceship earth. We are truly vital specks of loving stardust evolving toward a destiny that we help to shape.

How do I love thee? Let me count the ways.
I love thee to the depth and breadth and height
My soul can reach, when feeling out of sight
For the ends of Being and ideal Grace.
- Elizabeth Barrett Browning

The great poets have reminded us that a loveless life is, in fact, a living death. It is the spirit of love that actually makes our life "heavenlike". The unloving life without care, attachment or devotion often results in the personal hell of despair and purposelessness. Without love, we are nothing but unattached, lonely beings. But if we involve ourselves with others through care, help and nurturance, we may also realize personal growth, renewal and more zest in living.

+ GOOD-HEARTEDNESS +

Practice good-heartedness towards all beings.
Be loving and compassionate
no matter what others may do to you
...this is true spirituality.
-Tibetan Book of Living and Dying

+++ A LOVABLE DOG+++

Welcomes you with joy.

Accepts you just as you are.

Cheers you up.

Reflects the care of its master.

Protects you when necessary.

Keeps you in real touch with nature.

Helps you walk and keep fit.

Knows when to play and when to obey.

Makes you feel wanted and needed.

Delights in being petted, brushed and groomed.

Actually enjoys listening to you.

Makes you laugh and feel better.

Can help you live a more full and happy life.

Is a great companion you can always count on!

-A Personal Survey-

This is the time to stop and reflect on your own life and loving care by completing the following sentences as rapidly as you can. Express the first thought or feeling that comes to your mind. Make additional comments as needed.

1. My first experience with loving care was-
2. My first true love was -
3. If I love others as myself -
4. Mature love is -
5. Some of the risks of love I have experienced are -
6. I could improve my love life by -
7. At times it is difficult for me to give loving care because -
8. If we truly love and care for ourselves -
9. I have been greatly nurtured by -
10. The spirit of love -

7

---- PRAYER and MEDITATION ----

More things are wrought by prayer than this world dreams of.
-Alfred, Lord Tennyson

Many persons find renewed strength and purpose through prayer, meditation, yoga and other forms of contemplation. Prayer consists of the belief in a greater God or creative life force beyond ourselves which may be available to help us. Through such means as petition, adoration or self-reflection, we attempt to communicate with the divine in ourselves, nature and the broader universe of which we are a part.

For some persons, church affiliation provides religious identification and opportunity for communal prayer, support and other renewing experiences. Wherever it may occur, the psychological effects of prayer are such that once one's aspirations are clearly formulated and *asserted*, personal behavior tends to change accordingly. As Soren Kieregaard has aptly stated, "Prayer does not change God, but changes him who prays."

The power of prayer has been acknowledged by people in all cultures in many different ways. Where prayer is positive and contemplative, it often answers the need of the individual for self-expression and direction in life. Some prayers also provide reassurance and comfort as needed.

God grant me the serenity to
accept the things I cannot change,
courage to change the things I can,
and the wisdom to know the difference.
-Reinhold Niebuhr

There is an intrinsic drive toward wholeness and integration within the unconscious psyche of all people during prayer and meditation. Perhaps the most feasible form of self-renewal available to everyone is meditation. Through personal contemplation and focused centering on sensory and reflective encounters with your inner Self, you can transcend mundane concerns. Transcendence means getting "out of" oneself by attempting to open and expand one's conscious mind. Meditative prayerfulness is a feeling of communion with the universal creative force which can result in profound personal feelings of self-renewal.

As we thinketh in our heart so are we.
-Romans 12:12

Meditation is deep continued thoughtful reflective dialogue between your creative Self and the "Spirit of Life" or "God" within you. The Self is an all inclusive term that embraces your whole living organism; it contains the inherited dispositions and totality of all past life and is also the fertile soil from which all future life will spring. The inner meditative focus on affirmations, sounds, symbols, ideas and supra-personal images in the unconscious mind can have transformational power on the life of the individual - resulting in insight, enlightenment, holistic health, serenity and the self-actualization of unique potentialities.

I can pass from the happiness of knowledge and virtue
to the eternal calm and joy and peace of the Spirit
when I become one with the highest Self
and with all beings.
-Bhagavad-Gita

Very little of our lifespan is spent in directed conscious activity. Our focused awareness is similar to the small tip of an iceberg floating in a deep ocean. Most mental and instinctual human functions occur through unconscious body-mind processes. At times, they emerge from a dynamic psyche as dreams, desires, intuitions and other forms of uniquely creative acts. St. Augustine admonished us "to seek not abroad but to turn back into thyself for in the inner person dwells the truth." Meditative prayer and affirmation enables us to channel these powerful re-creative forces for health and wholeness.

Through meditation, we can invite the spirit of life to prevail in our hearts and minds. By being receptive to the mysterious powers within us, we can open ourselves to the fullness of life and healing by love and care. For example, through meditative identification with other forms of life and cultures we can leave our immediate selfishness behind and move toward fuller humanness and oneness.

Respect all life. Respect the Self.
Respect all people.
Respect the Creative Spirit.
Respect balance and harmony.
-Hopi Meditation

There are many forms of meditation. Through passive silent meditation, we do nothing to activate the mind or emotions and make no attempt to judge or analyze. With humble silence and relaxation, we can shift our attention from the surface aspects of life to the depths of our being wherein we regenerate ourselves both physiologically and psychologically. Scientific studies have shown that silent meditation results in a hypometabolic state with quiescence of the sympathetic nervous system which can lead to better physical and mental health.

Other forms of meditation include direct focused contemplation of such natural objects as flowers, trees, rocks, food and light. We can also meditate while focused on beautiful statues or other forms of art, such as symbolic pictures or photographs. Active meditation and reflection can even occur during creative physical activities like dance, painting, golf and fascinating work.

For example, many persons practice integrated forms of body, muscle and breath control through the regular use of simple calisthenics, yoga or stretching exercises. A good way to begin without great exertion of effort is as follows:

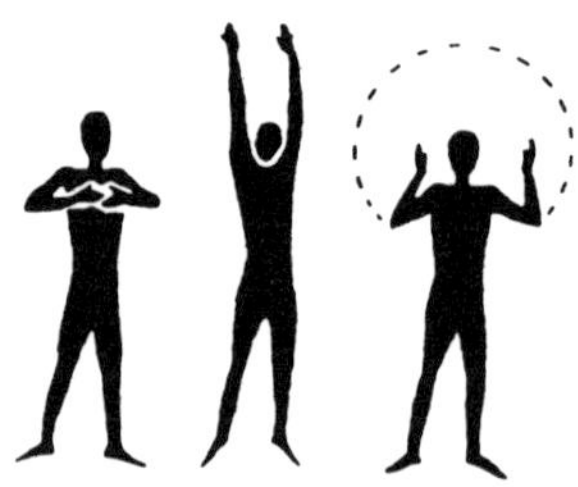

1. Stand up straight, in a balanced position, with palms flat on chest.
2. Slowly and *deeply* inhale as you raise your hands over your head, fingers outstretched, standing on tiptoes.
3. Slowly exhale as you bring your arms down in a semicircle and return hands to chest.
4. Repeat six times, breathing ever more deeply and slowly.

Let the words of my mouth and the meditation of my heart be acceptable in thy sight, O Lord, my rock and my redeemer.
-Psalms 19:14

Auditory meditation requires that we sit quietly and attempt to identify with certain sounds such as tranquil music, the ocean, trickling water or other rhythms - including our own deep breathing. Another simple and common form of auditory meditation is concentration on the slow, repetitious, rhythmic qualities of one's own voice in affirmation, song or chant. Even the constant repetition of words such as *joy, God, love, peace*, one's own name or the ancient *ohm* sound (which symbolizes universal life and energy) can have profoundly positve effects on the subconscious mind and body of the meditator. These meditations can be done by sitting confortably in a chair, on the floor or on a pillow.

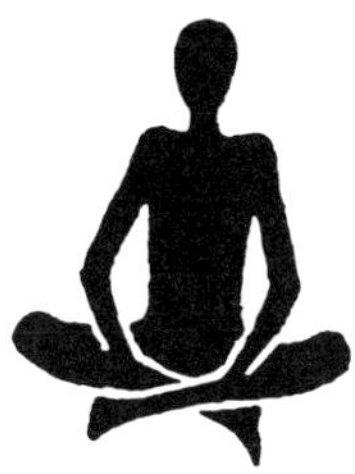

**Breath* - Begin by relaxing yourself through slow deep breathing. Silently count 20 deep breaths.

* *Flower* - Place a single flower in a vase before you. Carefully observe it and meditate on its beauty. Close your eyes and imagine a similar flower on a bush slowly opening itself to the sun in the morning. Re flect on the changing image of the flower.

* *Bread* - Hold fresh bread in your hand. Slowly break the bread and observe its texture. Close your eyes and smell it. Take a piece in your mouth and meditate on its taste and texture.

* *Music* - Play a favorite musical recording that you can "dream to." Place a lighted candle before you and concentrate on the flickering flame as you give yourself to the music.

Sound sleep by night; study and ease together mix'd; sweet recreation; and innocense, which most does please with meditation.
-Alexander Pope

Prayer and meditation can have profound healing effects. It has long been known that prayerful meditation has a positive healthful effect on the supplicating person; this has been attributed, in part, to psychological changes in self-esteem and acceptance. But it is only recently that the positive healing effects of prayer on other persons has been carefully studied and reported in scientific and medical journals. A review of this research has been published as *Healing Words* by Larry Dossey, M.D. who served as chairperson of the National Institutes of Health Office of Alternative Medicine.

In summary, in most studies, religious practice and meditation have significant positive effects on health. For example, eliciting the relaxation response alone, through prayer or any other means, reduced pain between 70 and 90% of the time. Coronary patients who were prayed for were five times less likely than controls to require antibiotics and three times less likely to develop pulmonary complications. Other serious medical conditions, such as cancer, have also been ameliorated.

Other profound effects of meditative states have been reported by psychologists and poets. The psychologist, William James, has described these as states of "transcendent wonder associated with absolute clearness of mind." The great poet, Alfred Lord Tennyson, was able to induce this state of being by repeating his name silently until his individuality seemed to dissolve and fade away into boundless being which he could only feebly describe:

Moreover, something is or seems,
that touches me with mystic gleams,
Like glimpses of forgotten dreams-
Of something felt, like something here;
Of something done, I know not where;
Such as no language may declare.

It appears that every person can profit from some form of earnest prayer or meditation which are most effective when used in conjunction with other healthful practices. But all people must develop their own distinctive styles based on their unique needs and experiences. Successful prayerful meditation helps to improve one's life and feelings of peace and contentment.

- A Personal Survey -

This is the time to stop and reflect on your own life of prayer and meditation by completing the following sentences as rapidly as you can. Express the first thought or feeling that comes to your mind. Make additional comments as needed.

1. Prayer and meditation -
2. Sometimes I have prayed -
3. A good place for me to meditate is -
4. An answer to my prayers -
5. Studies of prayerful meditation -
6. I can best get into contact with my inner Self -
7. A successful form of meditation for me -
8. My problems with prayer and meditation -
9. If everyone would pray and meditate -
10. The power of prayer is expressed -

8

---- POSITIVE AFFIRMATONS ----

> ***If we are no more than worms in this universe***
> ***I do believe that I am a glowworm.***
> -Winston Churchill

An affirmation is a strongly asserted belief, usually expressed as a positive statement or declaration of intent to act in certain ways. Common examples are legal oaths of honesty or allegiance, social pledges, marriage vows, religious creeds and personal self-affirmations. Emerson wrote that *belief consists in accepting the affirmations of the soul* which usually emphasize profound commitments to deeply held values such as love, honor, faith, loyalty and hope. These are all fundamental complex beliefs which are uniquely interpreted to give a feeling of meaning and importance to our lives.

Hope Springs eternal in the human breast:
Man never is, but always to be blest.
The soul, uneasy, and confined to home,
Rests and expatiates in a life to come.
-Alexander Pope

Over millions of years, humans have slowly evolved and been guided by chance and knowledge to become aware of the almost unlimited power of the human mind and spirit to learn and create in accord with our dreams and aspirations. In order to pursue and realize happiness we must first affirm our beliefs as specific aspirations. Our aspirations are the thoughts or ideals which provide us with goals and directions. Positive affirmations of our beliefs and aspirations become intrinsic self-motivators.

When human aspirations are strongly affirmed in word and action they become transformational psychic forces that directly influence our behavior. We tend to act in accord with our beliefs and affirmations. It is mankind's fate to creatively struggle with the material and spiritual problems of the time. And the forever occuring personal demons of self-doubt, uncertainty, unworthiness, despair and anxiety remain to be confronted in our daily quests for wholeness and personal fulfillment. But through positive statements and assertions, we can affirm our lives willfully and move ourselves to constructive action.

Whether you think you will succeed or not, you are right.
- Henry Ford

The first step then, in realizing human potentialities, is to believe in the power within ourselves to change for the better. History is a record of the many accounts of persons who acted on that which they believed. This power of belief is noted in the comment of John Stuart Mill that *one person with a belief is equal to the force of ninety who only have interests.* Winston Churchill's resolute belief in the powers of his inner self and his unusual affirmation as a "glowworm" helped England cope with wartime difficulties and had a dramatic positive effect on world history.

I wish I would - I think I can - I believe I will - I knew I could!

The founding fathers of the United States of America were unusually positive and affirmative of their beliefs. Some of them, like Thomas Jefferson, credited Christian idealism and the French enlightenment with their philosophical ideas. Jefferson went on to draft the Declaration of Independence, which included the following revolutionary affirmation of human rights:

We hold these truths to be self-evident,
that all men are created equal, that they
are endowed by their Creator
with certain unalienable rights,
that among these are life, liberty
and the pursuit of happiness.

Most people strongly believe in and affirm their rights to life, liberty and the pursuit of happiness. However, affirmations alone are insufficient to enable us to realize them. We must be willing and able to transform our beliefs into practical goals and committed affirmative action. It is only through successful action and personal achievement that we eventually develop more positive self-regard, which further enables us to assume greater control over our actions.

First say to yourself what you would be;
and then do what you have to do!
- Epictetus

Thomas Edison believed that the genius of personal success was only *one percent inspiration and ninety-nine percent perspiration.* Undoubtedly, the most important single cause of personal success or failure is what we believe about ourselves and what we decide to do about it. Nothing is achieved without willful affirmation, determination, work and enthusiasm - but the starting point is to always believe in the transforming powers of one's inner self.

***I Believe I Am**
A unique and precious human being
My own best friend and my own worst enemy
A lovable and loving person
Capable of realizing my potential
Self-respecting
Responsible for my own behavior
Learning from my mistakes
Creating a joyful life
An important part of the universe!*

If we believe in our self-worth and capabilities, we can then proceed to accomplish what we strongly desire. Sometimes, we doubt ourselves to the extent that we truly become our own worst enemies. Even the most difficult goals can be realized if we are committed enough to take the first step of just beginning whatever may be required.

Then one careful step at a time will usually get us where we really want to go. Thomas Paine, an American revolutionary, said that *these are the times that try a man's soul,* but most persons could make the same assertion for their own time and place. Although we certainly go through trying times of constant change, every day is a challenge to the individual soul to affirm itself positively.

***Everyday is a wonderful new opportunity**
to love, to learn, to laugh,
to care, to create, and to celebrate
the joy of life!*

We have powerful psychological forces within our psyche, but it is up to us to employ them as needed. This can be done by asserting our personal affirmations through modes of speech, writing, body-mind exercises, prayer or meditation and other creative acts. Whatever form of willful action we take, it is important to recognize that, with continued practice, we are likely to get better and better.

It is also important to realistically recognize our limitations while, at the same time, willing ourselves to do whatever we can do - no matter how little it may be. Another early American statesman, Edward Everett Hale, expressed this belief as a powerful self-affirmation which remains in common use:

I am only one but still I am one.
I cannot do everything but still I can do something.
And because I cannot do everything
I will not refuse to do
the something that I can do.

We gradually learn to affirm ourselves and that for which we believe is worth living. To a large extent, our self-concepts and affirmations are shaped by our families and educational experiences. As they mature, all persons gradually develop their minds and distinctive talents in accord with their predispositions, interests and opportunities. The psychoanalyst, Rollo May, emphasizes that one of the most important things that happens in human thought is the self-affirmation *"I conceive - I can - I will - I am"* and that the affirmations *"I can" and "I will"* are the essential experiences of personal identity.

+BECOMING A PERSON+
I hear - and I attend
I see - and I remember
I feel - and I wonder
I care - and I affirm
I speak - and I relate
I reflect - and I understand
I love - and I transcend
I experience - and I act
and so do I become a person!

++++ WISE & WITTY AFFIRMATIONS ++++

I will let a smile be my umbrella.

If life gives me lemons I will make lemonade.

I hope to find happiness wherever I go instead of whenever I go.

When I am good to others I am best to myself.

I will keep my words gracious & tender
for tomorrow I may have to eat them.

Oh Lord, help me to keep my mouth shut when I am in deep water.

I shall not take myself too seriously for no one else does.

It is better for me to wear out than to rust out.

I will always find a helping hand at the end of my arm.

My real reward for having done something well is to have done it.

I wish to live in such a way that when I die
even the undertaker will be sorry.

- A Personal Survey -

This is the time to stop and reflect on your own life and positive affirmations by completing the following sentences as rapidly as you can. Express the first thought or feeling that comes to your mind. Make additional comments as needed.

1. I believe that I-
2. I wish I would-
3. I think I can-
4. I knew I could-
5. I admire-
6. I will-
7. I affirm my-
8. I would-
9. I respect-
10. I am-

9

---- GOOD HUMOR ----

A cheerful heart is good medicine, but a downcast spirit dries up the bones.
- Proverbs 17:22

It has been said that people are the only animals that can laugh at themselves. This is because we have gradually evolved a sense of humor which has enabled us to recognize and express ridiculous behavior in self and others. The creative pursuit of happiness involves good humor and laughter. People who cultivate a sense of humor in self and others usually find life more interesting, amusing and enjoyable. Humor is a marvelous human trait that helps bring joy and health. Joyful laughter also enables the human spirit to transcend sorrow and tribulation.

Humor is the distinctly human faculty of perceiving, thinking, speaking and writing what is amusing, ridiculous or funny. The primary purpose of humor is to decrease or relieve tension and anxiety. When we think of a favorite joke or funny situation, we actually produce special biochemicals in the brain and body, such as endorphins, which help us to relax and, if necessary, renew ourselves through an enhanced immune system. Laughing itself causes us to secrete hormones that rouse us to high alertness. As these biochemicals circulate in the blood they drive the laugh by stimulating the heart, other glands, breathing and the contraction of the arteries. A good laugh gives a hearty workout to practically every organ in the body.

By learning to laugh at our own silly actions, mistakes and humorous situations, we immediately reduce stressful reactions. It is good to learn to laugh at most of our own foolish mistakes -since most every one else will. Laughter is even being prescribed in hospitals with the use of clowns, music and other kinds of humor programs. Good humor can be hazardous to illness. It pays to remember that a smile is a good umbrella and that laugher can be powerful medicine!

Good humor is a tonic for mind and body.
It is the best antidote for anxiety and depression,
It attracts and keeps friends, It lightens human burdens.
It is the direct route to serenity and contentment.
-Graville Kleirser

***Happiness is a good martini, a good meal,
a good cigar and a good woman -or a bad woman-
depending on how much happiness you can take!***
- George Burns

Scientific research has shown that people who frequently smile and laugh actually have better health. In fact, a good laugh a day does help to keep the doctor away and contributes to a happy life and longevity. Because of this positive effect, laughter has been described as a form of "inner jogging" which stimulates the special sunshine within us to dispel sadness and frustration.

Laugh and the world laughs with you; weep and you weep alone.
-Ella Wheeler Wilcox

In this way, humor defuses sorrow and pain and eases the stress of daily life and existence. The deliberate recall of an amusing thought or situation often brings pleasant feelings and restores our healing powers. Without doubt, the inner chuckle can also brighten the day and open our minds to insightful thought and personal problem solving.

Most civilizations have valued the ability to identify and laugh at the absurdities of life and to apply these insights to personal and social improvement, thus contributing to their survival. Good humor helps to oil the wheels of life, to decrease friction and to keep society running smoothly. Whenever friendly humor is shared with other persons, through gags, pranks, witticisms, cartoons or theatrical comedy, it helps to put us at ease and to make us feel better.

+ THE ANATOMY OF HAPPINESS +

***Lots of truisms don't have to be repeated but there is
one that has got to be,
Which is that it is much nicer to be happy than
it is not to be.
And I shall even add to it by stating unequivocally
and without restraint
That you are much happier when you are happy
than when you ain't.***
- Ogden Nash

+++HUMOROUS INSIGHTS+++

I am an atheist, and I thank God for it!
-George Bernard Shaw

A person sometimes has a clear conscience
simply because his head is empty.
-Ralph Sackman

In Genesis it says it is not good for a man to be alone
but sometimes it can be a great relief.
-John Barrymore

Blessed are the young for they shall inherit the national debt.
-Herbert Hoover

When a man's dog turns against him it is time for a wife
to pick up her trunk and go home to mama.
-Mark Twain

An archeologist is the best husband any woman can have -
the older she gets, the more he is interested in her!
-Agatha Christie

The man who is always worrying whether or not his soul will be damned
generally has a soul that isn't worth a damn.
-Oliver Wendell Holmes

Nobody will ever win the battle of the sexes
because there's too much fraternizing with the enemy.
-Henry Kissinger

It is great to live with the saints in heaven,
but it is hell to live with them here on earth.
-Richard Cardinal Cushing

If humor is well expressed, through puns, proverbs, tales or satirical stories, the words and ideas can become more powerful representations of reality and may result in better understanding and dramatic changes in behavior.

Humorous songs and chants also have curative and restorative powers; for example, we may quickly alleviate the blues by singing joyful songs or jingles like *There isn't any trouble that won't vanish like a bubble if you only take the trouble just to S-M-I-L-E!* Such powerful thoughts are wonderful products of the human spirit and creative imagination.

King David and King Solomon
lived merry, merry lives
With many, many lady friends,
and many, many wives.
But when old age crept up on them,
with all its many qualms,
King Solomon wrote the Proverbs,
and King David wrote the Psalms.
-Anon

Skillful humor does spur the imagination and can be used to help us learn to cope more effectively by helping to increase cooperation and harmonious relations between groups of widely different people. Because a good sense of humor facilitates personal well-being and communication, it is something to be treasured and nurtured.

Although we are all born with a potential sense of humor, it is personally developed by family nurturing, conscious effort and numerous forms of multimedia. The smile of common joy from shared beliefs, endeavors and accomplishments helps to bind people together. Friendly humor helps to renew and recreate ourselves and others and contributes to the development of community.

Give me a sense of humor, Lord,
Give me the grace to see a joke,
To get some pleasure out of life
And pass it on to other folk.
-Anon

There are many things we can consciously do to improve our sense of good humor. Deliberately looking for humorous items in the news and media, such as personal notices, stories, jokes and comics is easy to do. Start a scrapbook of varied materials. Place cartoons and quips on the refrigerator or bulletin board at work. Send friends humorous cards for special events. Attend theatrical comedies. Give joke books, videotapes and recordings as gifts. But most important of all, determine to frequently share your good humor with family, friends and neighbors!

When we can begin to take our failures non-seriously,
it means we are ceasing to be afraid of them. It is of
immense importance to learn to laugh at ourselves.
-Katherine Mansfield

Life itself has been described as an ongoing pilgrimage of the spirit. It is a long tragic-comic journey from childhood innocence to youthful exuberance, adult certainty, middle age skepticism and elderly bewilderment. This journey includes many joys and sorrows, laughs and giggles - and lots of sour grapes.

Fortunately, as most people get older they also get happier if they have good health - and a little selective memory loss. Perhaps an old Scottish motto best advises us on how to travel our life journeys with the advice to laugh and *be happy while we're living for we're a very long time dead!*

+THE GOLDEN YEARS+
Old folks are worth a fortune: with silver in their hair,
gold in their teeth, stones in their kidneys,
lead in their feet and gas in their stomachs.
As soon as I wake, Will Power helps me get out of bed.
Then I go to see John.
Then Charley Horse comes along and when he leaves
Arthur Ritis shows up and stays the rest of the day.
After such a busy day, I'm really tired
and glad to go to bed - with Ben Gay!
But I thank my lucky stars that
I still have some teeth to chew with
and a good sense of humor
which helps me to keep my old friends.
-Anon

--- GOOD HUMOR ---

Creates joy and laughter.

Binds friends together.

Eases daily work and toil.

Elevates the spirit.

Strengthens family ties.

Calms the nerves.

Lessens conflict and hostility.

Challenges the mind.

Brightens dark days.

Helps heal old wounds.

Tantalizes the imagination.

Dispels despondency.

Stimulates insight.

Enriches the heart.

Promotes good health.

Benefits the soul.

Lengthens life.

A Personal Survey

This is the time to stop and reflect on your own life and good humor by completing the following sentences as fast as you can. Express the first thought or feeling that comes to your mind. Make additional comments as needed.

1. Good humor is -

2. Some things that make me laugh are -

3. One of my favorite jokes is -

4. A favorite comedian of mine -

5. Smiles -

6. When children laugh and giggle -

7. A humorous writer I enjoy reading is -

8. A funny comic strip I like is -

9. One of the silly things I have done is -

10. When I think of humorous things -

10

----- VISIONARY IMAGINATION -----

Where there is no vision, the people perish.
-Proverbs 29:18

Visionary imagination is the power to see something in the human mind which will have a profound effect on the person's future behavior. This creative power is most often used by a person to envision or picture something new or innovative in his or her mind. These powerful mental images are frequently received as some future idealistic change in the person or environment. Most persons can imagine some desirable physical changes in themselves or in their environment for which they wish to strive.

Our ideals are those ultimate aims or models of performance that we can create in our imaginations. Ideal images are not completely realistic, as they tend to portray concepts of perfection and wholeness which are seldom realized. But when we clearly picture our desires as ideal situations in our minds, it gives us pleasure and encouragement to change accordingly. Without personal and social vision of a desirable future we begin to languish and perish.

Homo sapiens is a unique species; it can envision its future, understand what is necessary to actualize it and then systematically proceed to imaginatively design and bring it into being. In the creation myths of many cultures, man has been bestowed with these god-like gifts to take dominion over the earth and all of its inhabitants. As the image of God with creative powers, we have actually become co-architects of the world in which we live.

God created man in his own image,
in the image of God created he him;
male and female created he them.
And God blessed them, and God said unto them,
...replenish the earth, and subdue it, and have dominion over
... every living thing that moveth upon the earth.
- Genesis 1:27-28

People experience vivid mental images during fascinating work or play, dreams, speculative contemplation, meditation, fantasy, sensory deprivation or illness. But it takes a sense of mission and strong personal determination to convert dreams to reality. It is the idealists and visionaries who have been foolish enough to throw caution to the wind and express their dreams and faith in some supreme deed, who have advanced mankind and enriched the world.

Hold fast to dreams
for if dreams die
life is a broken-winged bird
that cannot fly.
-Langston Hughes

Through creative imagination, we can envision ourselves in the process of growing, becoming and constructing. We can willfully develop and use this power to recreate ourselves, as well as our environment. A person who envisions things frequently becomes an innovative scientist, artist, revolutionary thinker, poet, controversial leader, dreamer, sage or prophet.

With imagineering and practical application, the visionary person may eventually become a creative genius. When human thought and action imaginatively and creatively apply knowledge and information, problems are solved, new products emerge and life is changed.

Imagination is more important than knowledge.
-Albert Einstein

The creative imaginations of scientists, artists and writers have given us much to enjoy. For example, Einstein relied primarily on the initial development of visual images and imaginative ideals before he began the rational mathematical analysis of available data. He also promoted the development of independent thinking and judgment, rather than the detailed acquisition of special knowledge.

Since then, an Imaginarium has been created at Stanford University and other places to explore the relationship between thinking, understanding and creativity. In the history of science, Einstein was not alone in his use of imagination to stimulate the mind and soul to innovative creativity.

Our Souls have sight of the immortal sea
which brought us hither,
can in a moment travel thither,
and see the children sport upon the shore,
and hear the mighty waters rolling evermore.
- William Wordsworth

Samuel Howe invented the sewing machine as a result of dream-like images. The chemist Friedrich Kekule discovered the molecular structure of benzene through several dreams. Thomas Edison constantly played with imaginative ideas until they evolved into experimental possibilities and finally resulted in the creation of the light bulb and numerous other practical things. A physiologist, Otto Loewi, conceived of the chemical transmission of nervous impulses in a dream state.

However, it is through poetic language and vivid artistic forms that the power of creative imagination is most widely seen. The evolution of powerful mental imagery is clear for all to see in the works of artists such as Leonardo Da Vinci, Michelangelo, Salvadore Dali and numerous others. The strange visions and daydreams of Robert Louis Stevenson gave rise to a number of famous books including *Dr. Jekyll and Mr. Hyde.* Guiseppe Tartini and many other musicians have also created great works from similar states of altered consciousness; John Lennon, for instance, was inspired to write the popular composition, *Imagine,* with these visionary lines:

Imagine all the people living life in peace-
you may say I'm a dreamer but I'm not the only one-
I hope someday you'll join us and the world will be as one.

Poets rely on visionary imagination to free the soul's creative power to enchant the human mind and body. Samuel Coleridge wrote the poem, *Kubla Khan,* after a dream. The ethereal poet, Kahlil Gibran, stated that imagination finds a road to the realm of the gods where the soul is liberated. William Wordsworth believed that imagination is but another name for absolute power, clearest insight, amplitude of mind and reason in her most exalted mood - and that it is imagination which enables us to comprehend different states of being.

Alfred, Lord Tennyson is recognized for his visionary poetry - such as the following excerpt from Locksley Hall, which helped to inspire the organization of the World Court and the United Nations.

PROPHECY

Men, my brothers, men the workers,
ever reaping something new:
That which they have done but earnest
of the things that they shall do:
For I dipt into the future, far as human eye could see,
Saw the vision of the world,
and all the wonder that would be...
In the Parliament of man, the Federation of the world.
Forward, forward let us range,
Let the great world spin forever
down the ringing grooves of change.
-Alfred, Lord Tennyson

Loren Eisley, an archeologist, has aptly described man as a "cosmic orphan symbol shifting magician" who is constantly being transformed through his novel ideas, images and their products. By creative imagination, we are also able to transcend ourselves and the world in which we live. Mankind continuously modifies itself, its culture and its physical environment through the never ending interplay of novel thoughts and symbolic images.

All civilizations and their artifacts are products of this never ending evolutionary process. Your mental images and visualizations of the kind of person you want to become and the kind of life you want to live have a powerful impact upon your behavior. The dreams of future possibilities spark the soul to creative endeavors.

It is the marriage of the soul with Nature
that makes the intellect fruitful,
brains that give birth to imagination...
We believe that the possibility of the future
far exceeds the accomplishment of the past.
We review the past with common sense,
but we anticipate the future with transcendental senses.
- Henry David Thoreau

By imagining our ideals and what we might yet become, we are actively constructing our happiness. Thomas Jefferson asserted that he liked the dreams of the future better than the history of the past because such dreams possess transformational powers. Fruitful imagination culminates in the practical realization of at least some of our ideals. All persons possess creative imagination, intuition and transformational powers, although they may be undeveloped or neglected. But every man and woman strives to rise above the mundane elements of his or her existence through dreams, fantasies and hopeful images of the future.

The great cellist, Pablo Casals, underscored the importance of learning that humans are uniquely creative marvels who have evolved over millions of years with no identical counterparts. As evolutionary creations of novel potentialities and possibilities for the future, the philosopher, Henri Bergson, advocated that we learn to use and directly channel the vital life forces within us to improve our own lives. In reality, your self image, your social image and the ever changing images in your mind, of the world about you, actually determine how you function in daily affairs.

Startling physical feats have been accomplished by persons who have purposely used positive mental imagery to improve their lives. Numerous athletes have been guided by mental imagery and rehearsal in record breaking performances. The careful mental rehearsal of social skills, good work habits, emotional states and other behaviors almost always has significant results. This unusual magic-like power of visionary mental imagery was aptly noted by William Shakespeare:

Such tricks hath strong imagination, that,
if it would but apprehend some joy it
comprehends some bringer of that joy.

Perhaps the most joyful illustration of the power of creative imagination is in the recovery from illness and the maintenance of good health. By a positive interpretation of thoughts and feelings, our mental images can initiate a flow of chemicals in our system that actually evokes a healing response within the mind and body. For instance, the writer, Norman Cousins, recovered from a serious degenerative disease by using a holistic health program consisting of laughter, music, and positive visualizations of body *re*generation.

Dr. Albert Schweitzer used a combination of Bach's music, purposeful mental imagery and medicine to recover from his own illness. Dr. Carl Simonton and other physicians have successfully helped cancer patients develop positive mental images of their white corpuscles and body processes to combat disease. Similar mind-body studies are now being conducted in other research centers.

As thoughts and the ideas of things are arranged in the mind,
exactly so are the modifications of the body
or the images of things arranged and connected in the body.
-Spinoza

Another striking example of the holistic power of visionary imagination is the recovery from a heart attack by the psychologist, Carl Jung. Near death and in a state of altered consciousness, Dr. Jung experienced several symbolic visions of the universe in which he was " thronged round with images of creation". He later described these visions as the most tremendous things he had ever experienced and said that they resulted in profound feelings of bliss and joy. After his recovery, he credited these experiences as reenergizing his life with a sense of wholeness which also stimulated his most fruitful work. Jung professed that all the works of humankind have their origin in the powers of creative imagination.

Visionary mental images are forms of creative awareness and healing power unlimited by time, space or place and are interconnected with our bodies, minds and spirits. By self-actualizing our creative imaginations, we can renew ourselves and become more whole, healthy and happy individuals. This requires a willingness to open ourselves to personal exploration through mind-body exercises, creative mental imagery and practical application. Accordingly, the power of human imagination can make us infinite through the positive expression of our creative potentialities. In this way, we continually recreate ourselves and contribute to the design of the greater universe of which we are a significant part.

Hold fast to the great image and all under heaven will come;
they will come but not be harmed, rest in safety and peace...
When the Way is put to use, it is inexhaustible!
-Tao Te Ching

~~~ ENVISIONING~~~

Purpose: This guided exercise in mental imagery will enable you to envision some of the more desirable qualities of your Self.

Procedure: Tape record this script with a soothing musical background. Sit or lie down in a relaxed position as you listen to the tape.

Relax and let your tensions drain away. Close your eyes, breathe slowly and deeply and let yourself be even more at ease. Now imagine that your creative energy is slowly flowing through your head and coming to rest in your mind's eye. You feel very relaxed and comfortable as creative energy begins to focus within your mind.

Now visualize yourself feeling good, capable and full of confidence. You are a good, capable and confident person! You are going to envision in detail some of the many good things you have already done or accomplished. Imagine yourself when you were a child, at a time you were feeling very good about something that you had done. See what you had been doing. Let yourself reexperience the good feelings of that time. Quietly enjoy this scene for a few moments.

* This time, visualize yourself as a teenager enjoying an accomplishment and being praised by family and friends. Feel the sense of joy and celebration.

* Now envision yourself as an adult, with a sense of great satisfaction for completing a job well done, even though no one else was fully aware of it. Reexperience what you were doing and your deep feelings of self satisfaction.

* Finally, Imagine some of the many positive creative potentialities within your Self that are still waiting to be realized. Envision yourself in the process of joyfully doing something you desire and hope for in the near future. Experience in detail this process of becoming and the accompanying intrinsic rewards.

Now listen to yourself and silently repeat these words of self assertion:

I am a good and capable person.
I am a unique person with special talents and potentialities.
I am an important part of the universe.
I am envisioning myself becoming more complete.
I am feeling joyfully contented and accomplished.

-A Personal Survey-

This is the time to stop and reflect on your own life and visionary imagination by completing the following sentences as rapidly as you can. Express the first thought that comes to your mind. Make additional comments as needed.

1. My imagination -

2. I dream about -

3. Sometimes I envision myself -

4. One of my favorite fantasies -

5. Visions -

6. Future possibilities -

7. A powerful visionary experience -

8. Prophets -

9. I can envision the world -

10. Ten years from now -

11

---- CREATIVE EXPRESSION ----

Creative art (whether the instrument of words she use, or pencil pregnant with ethereal hues) demands the service of a mind and heart.
-William Wordsworth

Creative expression is the attempt of the individual human psyche to realize its potentialities. Psychologically, humans are islands forever struggling to live with themselves and others. Much of our life and energy is actually spent in a silent but dynamic dialogue with our inner selves in the pursuit of our dreams, interests and creative inclinations. Whenever we express ourselves through art, music, song, dance, writing, cooking, hobbies or other recreative activities, we renew our vital spirits and help transform the world about us.

It also takes courage and effort to create because creativity is the process of bringing something new into being through encounter and engagement with your unconscious spirit - with all of its potentialities for becoming different. These creative encounters can occur as playful fantasy, imaginative reverie, meditation, the imagery of insightful intuitions and conscious choices. When creative inclinations and interests are actively pursued, they are usually self-fulfilling and satisfying.

Every person has unique talents, special interests and vast creative potentialities, but these transformational powers may be relatively undeveloped, neglected or deliberately thwarted by authoritarian pressures or demands. Although surrounded by creative artifacts, many persons are unconscious or unaccepting of their own creative talents and potentialities. We all need to become more aware that the uniquely creative force within us is the perpetual evolutionary drive toward novelty and possibility, which we can use and channel for our betterment.

- CREATIVITY -

I am the secret of perpetual youth,
the everlasting creator of life;
where I am not, death rages...
from the rock whereon I light,
new life begins to flow.
-Richard Wagner

Happiness lies in the joy of achievement and the thrill of creative effort.
-Franklin D. Roosevelt

Individual creative expression normally occurs with time, nurturance and encouragement of special interests and abilities. It requires personal courage to playfully explore new ways of thinking and acting without undue fear or rejection. These are the very characteristics that are generally found in young children before they are suppressed by cultural conditioning. But these restrictions are gradually overcome when the opportunity to joyfully express oneself occurs. Creative thinking and expression can also be developed and refined through deliberate effort, training and education.

Work and avocational pursuits also offer various challenges for creative expression. There are many forms of work and effort required in life. Much of our time is spent in doing mundane everyday things, such as cooking, cleaning and repairing, that are required to sustain life. We are also involved in work related tasks and activities that are not personally meaningful or fulfilling; however, even these tasks can offer some outlet for creative expression.

When work is freely undertaken, it reflects our interests and concerns. Most jobs present personal challenges to growth and self-expression. The early scientist-philosopher, Galen, noted that gainful work is nature's physician because the person so occupied tends to retain or regain self-respect and high morale. We give ourselves to work or play in varied degrees, depending on opportunity and circumstances.

Happiness has been described as a journey of creative effort that includes some attainment of those things for which we commit ourselves to work. Blessed are those fortunate persons who have found creative expression and self realization in their work. But invariably, we need to turn to play and recreation to adequately express our creative inclinations.

A little work, a little play to keep us going
-- and so, good-day!
A little warmth, a little light of love's bestowing
-- and so, good-night!
A little fun, to match the sorrow of each day's growing
--and so, good-morrow!
-George Louis Palmella

Studies show that the average American spends about 20 hours a week on leisure time activities, such as television, reading, walking, hobbies and other creative pursuits. Arts and crafts, sports, music and dramatic activities are the most common forms of creative expression. Active interests are intrinsically rewarding; play and fun expand our personal horizons and involve us in the larger world around us.

Thoughts are free and are subject to no rule -
and give birth to creative force.
-Paracelsus

Creative art is that in which the hands follow the head and the heart, bringing personal satisfaction. The glory of a pleasing painting, sculpture or other kind of art is not only that it is pleasurable to create, but that it can also immortalize the beauty of the moment and be inspirational to others in the future. Next to the beauty of nature, art is venerated for its magnificence and endurance.

Because of its immediate effect on us, music is often described as the supreme art. Songs frequently express our heartfelt dreams and desires, such as love and celebration. Listening to music also wards off boredom and anxiety and can enhance concentration and pleasurable experience.

Sing and dance together and be joyous.
-Khalil Gibran

When people sing and dance together, they share joy and fellowship. Music has been recognized as having celestial powers which can soothe the body, calm the mind and bring harmony to the community. People are also moved and inspired by music which touches their hearts and souls. The music of the spheres is like the beating of a heart; its rhythm repeats the greater harmony of which we are a part.

We laugh, we cry, we live, we die,
we dance, we sing our song
to something to which we can belong.
-Shelley Jackson Denham

The creative human spirit is also expressed through fantasy and daydreams. Fantasy is imaginative speculation about something of concern. It begins with the free association and exaggeration of facts and information. Productive fantasy occurs when a valued product emerges from this creative process. Fantasy is powerfully expressed in artistic and musical productions such as Walt Disney productions, cartoons, myths and fairy tales. Dr. Seuss books, science fiction, and romance novels are all popular literary examples of the appeal of creative fantasy as a joyful escape mechanism in everyday life.

Time and experience is unceasing creation,
the uninterrupted up-surge of novelty.
-Henry Bergson

Imaginative play and make-believe facilitate language development and the ability to categorize and think. Constructive fantasy, such as make-believe and "pretend" games, contributes to the development of higher order language and thinking skills and makes learning more pleasurable and productive. Legends and fairy tales are traditional examples of creative expression through which we can explore our thoughts and feelings. Television soap operas are also ever-present reminders of the power of fantasy in our lives.

The creative spirit is expressed through our individual personalities and talents which enrich and transform our lives. We are surrounded by the results of human creativity portrayed in the inventions and products of civilization, which include everything from soaring cathedrals to nuclear weapons. Our continuing challenge is to learn to joyfully express our creative inclinations in positive and constructive forms that will contribute to our personal development, as well as to the furtherance of humanity as a whole.

For ye shall go out with joy,
and be led forth with peace:
the mountains and the hills shall
break forth before you into singing.
-Isaiah 55:12

I am the CREATIVE SELF
that dwells in the heart
of every mortal creature.
I am the beginning,
the lifespan,
and the end of all.
Whatever in this world is powerful,
beautiful or glorious that you may know,
has come forth from a fraction
of my power and glory.

-Bhagavad Gita

- A Personal Survey -

This is the time to stop and reflect on your own life and creative expression by completing the following sentences as rapidly as you can. Express the first thought or feeling that comes to your mind. Make additional comments as needed.

1. My creative abilities -
2. Some of my talents include -
3. One of the things I have created -
4. I enjoy playing -
5. My hobbies -
6. A favorite form of recreation for me is -
7. It is fun to -
8. Some of my creative efforts enjoyed by others are -
9. A long time interest of mine is -
10. When I express myself creatively -

12

---- HEALTHY HABITS ----

The natural healing force within each one of us is the greatest force in getting well.
-Hippocrates

Good health is the result of harmony between a person's body, mind, spirit and soul. With inner harmony, our vital energy is balanced and renewed and we enjoy life more fully. Vitality is the essence of joyful being. The state of your health largely depends on your unique physical constitution, proper exercise and moderation in your personal behavior. To a considerable extent, the soundness of your body, mind and spirit is established through consistent practice of healthy habits. The father of medicine, Hippocrates, recognized that the most important factor in good health was how we utilize the natural healing force within us.

Healthy people are more optimistic about their lives and feel that they have more control over what happens to them. It is through our practice of healthy habits that we can nurture and direct the natural healing force within us. All persons must decide what is the best way for them to nurture this healing force which enables them to be healthy and happy. But there are general habits for maintaining good health that apply to all people. These include proper medical care, nutrition, rest, relaxation, hygiene, exercise and positive attitudes for dealing with pain, stress and disease.

Preventive medicine emphasizes the importance of early diagnosis and regular health checkups. It has been found that an ounce of prevention of disease is truly worth more than a pound of expensive cure or prolonged treatment. Periodic inoculations for contagious diseases, general cleanliness and good hygiene are all examples of highly effective preventive medicine. Also, almost all persons have some kind of physical and/or mental disability during their lives that could be minimized or compensated for with early awareness and systematic management. This requires that we consciously assume considerable personal responsibility for our own health and happiness by acting in a timely way and consistently, as needed.

Happiness is the result of a good conscience, good health, occupation, and freedom in all just pursuits.
-Thomas Jefferson

Establishing good eating and consumption habits is a difficult task for many people. The goal of course, is to ensure that we provide our bodies with required nutrients through appropriate amounts of balanced food groups. Recent studies make us increasingly aware of the importance of habituating ourselves to eating less, sticking with a diet low in fat and drinking at least eight glasses of water a day. Occasional controlled fasting may also be of value.

We know that we should eat to live and not live to eat - but for most people that is much easier said than done. However, considerable evidence exists that more and more people are eating more carefully as a result of education and conscious self-determination. Moderate use, or avoidance, of tobacco, alcohol and drugs also leads to a healthier life. Healthy consumption habits result in good digestion and proper nourishment of mind and body.

Everyone also needs regular and appropriate exercise. Civilization has considerably reduced physical activity and body movement to the extent that we may be endangered by loss of strength, endurance and flexibility. When coupled with inappropriate nutritional habits, this commonly results in serious overweight and muscular degeneration, contributing to coronary disease, stroke or other fitness problems. Varied exercise for as a little as 30 minutes three or four times a week (such as walking, aerobics, swimming, bicycling or weight lifting) is essential for all.

Numerous health and fitness clubs are now available to those who may need more personal attention and motivation. Vigorous periodic exercise can easily be supplemented daily with shorter stretching and tension reducing activities adaptable to every home or work situation. It is much better to gradually wear out from invigorating activity than to rust out from atrophy and disuse!

Blest, who can unconcernedly find hours,
days and years slide soft away,
In health of body, peace of mind,
quiet by day;
sound sleep by night; study and ease
together mixt; sweet recreation;
And innocence which most does please
with Meditation.
-Alexander Pope

+++ HEALTHWISE MAXIMS +++

He who laughs, lasts.

Eat not to dullness, drink not to elevation.

The best physicians are Dr. Diet, Dr. Quiet, and Dr. Merryman.

An apple a day keeps the doctor away.

A good wife and health are a man's best wealth.

Pleasant words are like honey, sweet to the soul and health to the body.

God heals, but the doctor takes the fee.

Three good meals a day is bad living.

Wish not so much to live long as to live well.

Early to bed and early to rise makes a person healthy, wealthy and wise.

No gains without pains.

Eat to live and not live to eat.

A person's spirit will endure sickness, but a broken spirit who can bear?

Nine men in ten are suicides.

Do all things in moderation.

There are no riches above a sound body.

Who is strong? - he who can conquer bad habits.

Adequate rest, sleep and relaxation are all subject to habitual control. Although many persons complain that they do not get enough sleep or rest, these problems can be lessened with deliberate effort. For example, when president Franklin D. Roosevelt realized he was unduly suffering from work stress and the ravages of poliomyelitis, he learned to renew his energy through short cat-naps. Relaxation techniques, such as a few minutes of sitting quietly and breathing deeply and systematically, can quickly calm and restore both mind and body.

When breathing exercises are used with soothing music, the sense of well being is further increased. But there is no substitute for the benefits of regular sound sleep, which is nature's basic way of restoring and balancing your life's energy. It is wise to pay attention to your body's demands to catch up on your sleep!

O magic sleep! O comfortable bird,
that broodes't o'er the troubled sea of mind
till it is hush'd and smooth.
-John Keats

Research has also shown that healthy people are more optimistic about their lives and feel that they have more control over what happens to them. Positive mental attitudes, such as self affirmation, good humor and meditation, activate the release of pain reducing biochemicals in the body, reduce depression, and increase creative flexibility of thought and action.

The prophet Isaiah (55:7-8) stated that when we let our inner *light break forth* by helping to feed the hungry and clothe the poor then *thine health shall spring forth speedily*. When we use our spiritual powers to help light the way for others, we also improve our own physical and mental health.

Look to your health; and if you have it, praise God,
and value it next to a good conscience;
for health is the second blessing
that we mortals are capable of;
a blessing that money cannot buy.
-Izaak Walton

Healing must be concerned with the soul as well as the body for no creature can be sound so long as the higher part of it is sickly.
- Pythagoras

Since our body functions tend to reflect the mental attitudes or moods on which we dwell, good mental hygiene significantly contributes to the alleviation of pain and distress. Peaceful contentment and happiness are derived not so much from pleasure as in rest from pain or extreme discomfort. Effective mental strategies for pain reduction consciously distract our focus from the discomfort of pain to more pleasurable or comfortable sensations. Listening to soothing music, recorded stories, guided mental imagery or the humorous experiences of good friends are all powerful distracters. So are television comedy, inspirational books or articles, favorite games and recalling happier times and events.

Fortunately, as creative beings, we can choose to act as we will - or to respond to momentary gratifications. Most people know what is best for them but it is often difficult to do what might be good for them. We all succumb to temptation at times, but the consequences are insignificant if we maintain healthy habits over the long run. An effective way of establishing good personal habits is to carefully note and reward ourselves for systematic progress.

The starting point is to list and prioritize the habits we wish to develop. For instance, Benjamin Franklin listed temperance, moderaton, cleanliness, tranquillity, silence and order among other behaviors of real concern to him. Then he focused on accomplishing one for a week at a time - without total disregard for the others. He noted that when he concentrated on temperance in eating and drinking for a week, he was able to be more successful if he recorded his daily progress in a calendar book.

Although we are easily swayed and given to the folly of momentary pleasure, it is possible to learn from our mistakes and to improve ourselves. By conscientiously practicing and reinforcing healthy habits, we actively participate in becoming more happy and wholesome persons.

Save us, our compassionate Lord, from our folly by your wisdom,
from our arrogance by your forgiving love,
from our greed by your infinite bounty -
and from our insecurity by your healing power
- Muslim Prayer

- MAJOR DETERMINANTS OF HOLISTIC HEALTH -

CONSCIOUS EFFORT:

Love	**Prayer & Meditation**	**Compassion**
Affirmation	**Positive Imaging**	**Good Humor**
Exercise	**Nutrition**	**Hygiene**
Music	**Art**	**Dance**

ECOLOGICAL DETERMINANTS:

Pollution	**(air, water, atmosphere)**
Electromagnetic fields	**(light spectrums, radiation, space-time)**
Social Disorganization	**(stress, overpopulation, crime)**

BIO-MEDICAL DETERMINANTS:

Molecular genetics (DNA)

Hormonal Regulation (testosterone, serotonin, epinephrene, etc.)

Medication

Surgical Intervention

SUB-CONSCIOUS FACTORS:

Cultural Conditioning and Value Systems

Subliminal motivation

Universal Mind

+++SELF RELAXATION+++

Purpose: Using your vital energy to deeply relax yourself.

Procedure: Read and tape record your own voice for use as needed

Sit in a comfortable position. Close your eyes and sit quietly for a moment. Now make a fist of your right hand. Make it as tight as you can - tighter and tighter! Feel the tension all the way up through your arm! Now let go! Relax your fist and arm and feel the tension draining away- it is a good feeling. Now clench your left fist as tight as you can. Tighter! OK, let go and relax your entire fist and arm. Shift your attention to your shoulders and neck muscles. Tense them up. Shrug your shoulders and then really tighten up. Hold the tension and count slowly to five. OK, let go and relax! breathe deeply and slowly count to ten as you drain off all the tension from your neck, shoulders and arms. Feel those muscles relax.

Now get a picture of yourself in your mind as you begin to tighten your entire body. Clench your fists. Tighten your arms. Tighten your neck - now your shoulders. Now imagine your whole body as tense and heavy. Count to five as you imagine yourself getting tighter. Hold it for a minute! OK, let go, breathe deeply as you count to ten and relax your fist, your arms, your neck, your shoulders and your entire body. Feel the energy circulating and nourishing your entire system. Breathe even more deeply as you lightly clasp your hands together over your abdomen. Become aware of the warmth of your body and the rhythmic rise and fall of your abdomen. Let yourself become aware of the wonderful harmonious workings of your body, mind and vital spirit.

Now quietly imagine your vital energy beginning to renew your entire system. Feel calm, comfortable, light and refreshed. Slowly begin to feel the flow of vital creative energy to your head and picture it as a lightly glowing star in your mind's eye. As it centers in your mind, become aware of the quiet healing and regenerating power emanating from this creative source within you. Feel good and renewed! Keep your eyes closed. Remain relaxed but quietly stand erect with your hands at your sides. Slowly raise your hands up over your head as you tilt your head back and stretch on your toes. Imagine your healing energy now encircling your entire body and revitalizing you as you peacefully move through the day ahead.

- A Personal Survey -

This is the time to stop and reflect on your own life and healthy habits by completing the following sentences as rapidly as you can. Express the first thought or feeling that comes to your mind. Make additional comments as needed.

1. My general health is -

2. One good healthy habit of mine is -

3. The best diet for me consists of -

4. The exercise I enjoy most is -

5. Some foods that tend to upset me are -

6. I last saw my physician for -

7. A good tension reduction exercise for me is -

8. I feel most energetic -

9. What pains me the most is -

10. I can usually cope with stress by -

13

---- SELF EXPECTATIONS ----

The purpose of life is to be that self which one truly is.
-Soren Kierkegaard

Most people expect to be happy and successful in their lives but they are not sure how to get there! Personal happiness depends upon the ability to successfully achieve our goals and aspirations. This assumes, of course, that we do have reasonable self-expectations and a plan and intention to work for their realization. But setting appropriate goals and expectations, planning how to achieve them and working to accomplish them require insightful self-knowledge and dedication.

Accordingly, the major requisite for becoming happy and successful is to believe that one's inner Self has the spirit and potentiality for achieving personal dreams and expectatons. If we are convinced that we are fundamentally good, sound and capable persons, we tend to act in accord with these positive self-concepts. However, the actual achievement of our self-expectations requires other willful qualities, personal habits and character strengths. These qualities include:

Self-knowledge and understanding **of strengths and limitations.**
Self-determination, **reliance and will to succeed.**
Self-discipline, **control, evaluation and regulation of work and effort.**
Self-responsibility **for one's behavior and actions.**
Self-respect and recognition **of personal accomplishments.**

Throughout the ages, man has been challenged to *know himself* as the most essential step in acquiring knowledge and understanding. To truly "know thyself" is a difficult task of developing awareness of our potentialities for becoming a unique person. This requires the willingness to search within ourselves to discover whatever special predispositions, abilities, talents, skills, interests and values we may possess and how they might best be used.

This above all: to thine own self be true,
and it must follow, as the night the day,
thou canst not then be false to any man.
-William Shakespeare

Self-knowledge also requires the courage to realistically acknowledge personal limitations and shortcomings and to attempt to balance them with strengths, dreams and aspirations. Self-expectations are derived from self-knowledge and understanding, with the eventual hope that their realization will result in joy and satisfaction.

Reasonable self-expectations provide us with meaningful goals for living and becoming more complete and happy persons. But our dreams and aspirations should also motivate us to do our very best.

A man's reach should exceed his grasp, or what's a heaven for?
-Robert Browning

One's true Self also consists of those qualities of a person which uniquely distinguish individual character and personality. These qualities include the sum of our inherent genetic traits plus social experience and conditioning - with great potentialities to thought and action, of which we are only dimly aware. One's inner Self contains a wealth of unconscious wisdom and human potential awaiting the dawn of creative exploration and development.

The Self then is the center of your earthly existence and the basic source of your continual striving to become a whole and healthy person. It is the integrated core of your mind, body and soul, which is reflected in the distinctive spirit of your personality. Although each of us is a mystery of unlimited potential, never to be fully understood by introspection or analysis, we can become more consciously aware of who and what we are. Through such experiences as education, contemplation, study, work, effort and intuitive reflection, it is possible to develop meaningful expectations and resolutions to direct and improve our lives.

What is a man anyhow? What am I? What are you?...
I know I am solid and sound:
I know I am deathless,
I know that I am august:
I exist as I am - that is enough;
One world is aware and by far the largest to me,
and that is myself!
- Walt Whitman

+ SELF ADAGES +

If you don't know where you are going
you are bound to get lost along the way.

Depend not on another, but lean instead on thyself.

True happiness is born of self-reliance.

There are three things extremely hard: steel, a diamond,
and to know oneself.

The greatest conqueror is he who conquers himself.

He that would please all and himself too,
undertakes what he cannot do.

Fools laugh at others; wise men at themselves.

Search others for their virtues, thyself for thy vices.

Wink at small faults - remember thou hast great ones.

He that cannot obey cannot command.

If you love yourself overmuch, nobody else will love you at all.

Well done is better than well said.

The man who aims at nothing is almost sure to hit it.

The desire accomplished is sweet to the soul.

Reasonable self-expectations, resolutions and efforts alone do not necessarily overcome bad habits, such as procrastination and disorganization, which may hinder our efforts to succeed. Self-discipline is the essential factor required for real success. For example, systematic self-evaluation and regulation of your own behavior can significantly improve performance of most tasks. Merely writing down your expectations with a sensible step-by-step plan for getting there, usually leads to success if honestly implemented, critically evaluated and carefully self-reinforced along the way. Constructively critical self-observation, correction and proper practice almost always result in accomplishment!

Self-discipline is easy when there is vision of the highest.
- Yoga Sutra

Without such self-discipline and control, we become overly dependent on others and may be easily manipulated or misguided. The person who lacks self-discipline becomes a pawn because of his poor habits, which then invites control by others. Eventually, the unruly child or adult is forcibly restrained and the person who fails to discipline himself to the demands of the job or social situation is restricted or removed by others.

When personal discipline and responsibility is lacking, the person becomes a slave to the passions of the moment which undermine willful self-detemination. Such emotionally unstable persons are easily frustrated and seldom happy. Self-reliance and control require that we be honest and true to ourselves in searching for our mistakes and striving for self-improvement.

Wise persons know they are bound to err and fall short of their expectations at times. But they have learned to adapt as needed. A good conscience and self-esteem help us to appropriately judge our own misdeeds, correct mistakes, forgive our errors and proceed to try again. The person who has learned to control his own tongue and temper, to regulate his work and leisure time and to assume responsibility for his actions has few sorrows or regrets in life.

A man without self-control is as defenseless as a city with broken down walls.
- Proverbs 25:28

No person realizes all of his or her human possibilities. Indeed, even under the best of circumstances, a person's vast potential remains somewhat of a mystery to self and to others. Robert Louis Stevenson wrote that to be what we truly are and to become what we can is our basic purpose in life. President Theodore Roosevelt expanded this concept by challenging us to do what we can *with what we have, where we are!* Certainly we are all capable of growing and becoming much more fulfilled than we now are.

Man is happy only in his aspiration to the heights; when he attains his goal, he cools and longs for other distant flights.
- Kahlil Gibran

The person who consciously determines to develop his or her self as much as possible does help to shape the future - and such individuals are usually happier than those whose lives are largely managed by others. The value of deciding what to do with our own lives has long been championed in American folk songs and modern music. For instance, some of the lyrics in *Life is a Song Worth Singing* are: *"Only you generate the power to decide what to do with your life - You're a fool if you think you're helpless; you control what to do with your life!"*

By assuming self-responsibility and self-determination, we can then take appropriate steps to acquire the knowledge, understanding and skills necessary to create more meaningful and fulfilling lives. Faith in the transforming power of our real selves revitalizes our spirits to love and care, to affirm and to imaginatively create a more harmonious and joyful existence. The successful pursuit of happiness results from a habitual life style of self-reliance that enables us to finally achieve most of our personal aspirations and expectations.

- Me and Myself -

I have to live with myself and so I want to be fit for myself to know.
I don't want to stand with the setting sun
and hate myself for the things I've done.
I never can hide myself from me,
I know what others may never know,
I see what others may never see.
So whatever happens I want to be
Self-respecting and conscience free.
- Anon

WHAT IS SUCCESS?

To laugh often and much.

**To win the respect of intelligent people
and the affection of children.**

**To earn the appreciation of honest critics and
endure the betrayal of false friends.**

To appreciate beauty.

To find the best in others.

**To leave the world a bit better, whether by a healthy child,
a garden patch, or a redeemed social condition.**

**To know even one life has breathed easier
because you have lived.**

This is to have succeeded.

- Ralph Waldo Emerson

- A Personal Survey -

This is the time to stop and reflect on your own life and self-expectations by completing the following sentences as rapidly as you can. Express the first thought or feeling that comes to mind. Make additional comments as needed.

1. What I most expect of myself is -
2. Some of my strengths are -
3. Some of my limitations are -
4. What I excel at is -
5. My major self-control problem is -
6. I plan -
7. Sometimes I have fooled myself by -
8. My sense of self-esteem is -
9. I have had difficulty with -
10. What I value most -

14

-----CELEBRATING COMMUNITY-----

Behold, how good and pleasant it is to meet together in fellowship.
-Psalm 133:1

One of the great joys in life is the celebration of kindred hearts and souls in the interdependent community of love and fellowship. We need each other. We live, love, learn and grow only to the extent that we become meaningfully involved with other people. By relating to others in the shared community of family, friends, neighbors and earthly travelers, we can best meet our common needs and interests. Significant others in community are those friends, lovers or family members who try to understand us and accept us for what we are and might become. We share ourselves and our innermost thoughts with them in a mutual compact of protection and encouragement.

Our very survival depends on the quality of care and nurturance we provide each other in our rapidly growing global community. Only through cooperative endeavors can we successfully cope with the traditional scourges of mankind, such as famine, war, disease, pestilence and rapidly emerging population and pollution problems. We now know that everything we do as individuals affects the entire global family of which we are a critical part.

When we become significantly involved with other persons, we help and care for them and grow in the process of contributing to the common good. This requires empathy for others, personal awareness and sensitivity. Most importantly, it involves identification with other persons through empathetic understanding of mutual interests and concerns. It also requires the give and take of compromise and personal sacrifice when needed. Such relationships are not easily begun or sustained.

+Friendship's Road+
Friendship is a chain of gold
shaped in God's all perfect mold.
Each link a smile, a laugh, a tear,
a grip of the hand, a word of cheer.
No matter how far, or heavy the load-
sweet is the journey on friendship's road.
-J.B. Downie

The universally accepted guideline in establishing good interpersonal relationships continues to be to treat others as you would want them to treat you. When we hurt or wrong another person, we also harm ourselves. The reward of unselfishness is intrinsic satisfaction and personal growth, as expressed in adages such as: "I know a man, they thought him mad, the more he gave, the more he had." Buddha suggested it is best to return love and good to the person who foolishly does wrong, since we must live with the consequences of our own behavior. Our rewards are especially gratifying when we partake in the mutual give and take of fellowship and community.

You get more joy out of giving joy to others and should put a good deal of thought into the happiness you are able to give.
-Eleanor Roosevelt.

We are what we do, and what we become in life depends on our thoughtful consideration of self and others. By providing helpful love and care to all things we encounter, we enrich the community and world in which we live. Improving the general welfare of the global community is the inevitable challenge of humans, the success of which depends on the ability to develop empathy with fellow beings experiencing similar plights. And empathy for others only emerges from the developing awareness of mutual interests and values - such as the recognition that unregulated use of forests, land, water and other natural resources results in worldwide strife and pollution, affecting all living things.

With empathy and greater understanding of our mutual concerns, the possibility of cooperative rational *problem-solving* dramatically increases. It is essential therefore that we cultivate the values of kindness, empathy, help and consideration in ourselves and others, since the kind of loving care and nurturance that is shared eventually affects the entire world. In order to realize our own potentialities, we must work harmoniously with others. Whatever we do, our personal destinies will forever remain intertwined with what happens everywhere.

May we be inspired to bring our gifts of
love and service to the altar of humanity.
And may we know once again that we are not
isolated human beings but connected, in mystery and miracle,
to the universe, to community and to each other.
-Anon

Cooperate and there will be no harm,
only happiness, order and peace.
-Tao 35

Nevertheless, it is a hard task to recognize common interests and values, and even more difficult to fairly share whatever sacrifices real solutions may require. When a person finally realizes what should be done for the common good, but deliberately continues to act in highly selfish ways, the potentiality of tragically destructive evil may become a frightening reality. If not suppressed, such amoral anti-social behavior can undermine the just community and society itself.

The alternative to the totalitarian state
is the cooperative community.
-Norman Thomas

The noted historian, H.G. Wells, concluded that human history becomes more and more a race between education and catastrophe. Wells felt that all educational institutions must begin to teach global problems and interests, together with possible lawful solutions - or humankind would be destroyed by its own ignorance and stupidity. Similarly, Albert Einstein proposed that if we are to overcome our prejudices and destructive tendencies, we must also learn to become critical thinkers capable of exercising independent judgment on governmental and international issues.

History provides us with records of human success and failure, from which we should learn to not repeat our mistakes. Science enables us to use objective methods and facts for creating new technologies. But our ultimate goals and visions of what we hope to individually and collectively become are formulated from dreams, aspirations and longings of the human soul. True individual happiness without self-control, rational concern and proper care of others is an impossible state of being.

The goal of human existence is to establish a community
of free and happy human beings who by constant
inward endeavor strive to liberate themselves from
the inheritance of anti-social and destructive instincts.
-Albert Einstein

-MARK TWAIN ON MORAL & ETHICAL BEHAVIOR-

Always do right - this will gratify some and astonish the rest.

Christianity is a good and gentle religion - but inconvenient!

Such is the human race - often it does seem such a pity that Noah and his party did not miss the boat!

Be virtuous and you will be eccentric.

All I care to know is that a man is a human being - that is enough for me; he can't be any worse.

Let us consider that we are all partially insane - it will explain us to each other.

Get your facts first and then you can distort them all you want.

From his cradle to his grave a man never does a single thing which has any first and foremost object but one - to secure peace of mind and spiritual comfort for himself.

It is curious that physical courage should be so common in the world and moral courage so rare.

Loyalty to the petrified opinion never yet broke a chain or freed a human soul.

If Christ were here there is one thing that he would not be - a Christian.

Let us live our life in such a way that when we die even the undertaker will be sorry.

The Self is largely determined by social factors and reflects both personal and cultural concerns. Cultures define values, norms and goals for the continued survival of civilization. These beliefs provide social guidelines for ways of acting within the community. The continually evolving rules of law and custom have considerable effect on human behavior. But individual actions are primarily motivated by our intrinsic interests, which reflect particular personal talents and inherited potentialities. What kind of persons we finally become actually depends on the choices we make as individuals, even though we are greatly influenced by our culture, community and genetic endowments.

The good man does not grieve that other people do not recognize his merits. His only anxiety is lest he should fail to recognize theirs.
-Confucius

Our own interests are usually best served through a combination of intimate personal relationships balanced with broader social commitment and involvement. Norman Vincent Peale was convinced that happiness never comes if it is a goal in itself, since real happiness is a by-product of commitment to worthy causes. By caring enough to participate with others in community service improvement organizations and projects, we expand the range of our own opportunities for growth and possibilities for happiness.

In the words of Winston Churchill, *we make a living by what we get, but we make a life by what we give.* For example, volunteer work with youth gangs, clubs, schools, the disabled or elderly all help to improve the quality of community life. So too does taking personal responsibility for joining self-help groups, such as Alcoholics Anonymous and many others, which bring people together for special kinds of mutual help and support.

Lives of great men remind us
we can make ourselves sublime,
and, departing, leave behind us
footprints on the sands of time.
Footprints, that perhaps another
sailing o'er life's solemn main,
a forlorn and shipwrecked brother,
seeing, shall take heart again.
-Henry Wadsworth Longfellow

The direct object of government is the happiness of the people.
-James Madison

Improving all parts of government, including the rules and regulations under which we live as civilized persons, is only possible through responsible citizen involvement. Thomas Jefferson said that in order to accomplish our constitutional goals and declarations, it may be necessary to make revolutionary changes in our government every twenty years or so! Martin Luther King, Jr. held that we should use peaceful means to *hew a stone of hope out of the mountain of despair.*

The most constructive way to pursue and achieve our happiness is by free and democratic participation in the never-ending process of self-development and realization - including voting for better government and societal improvement. To choose not to vote or exercise rights of citizenship is to place ourselves at risk of being increasingly controlled and directed by others who may act contrary to our personal interests and those of the general welfare. Through cooperative efforts, we can best realize the fruits of our labor and celebrate accordingly.

There is nothing better for a man, than that he should eat, and drink, be merry and enjoy the good of all his labour - it is the gift of God.
-Ecclesiastes 3: 8-15

The step-by-step achievement of our goals and aspirations calls for joy and celebration. During special events and holidays, we celebrate events that mark our personal progress along life's journey. It is celebration in the joy of our personal existence, the fellowship of community and the process of becoming that bring us happiness. We should also continually celebrate the ongoing creative process within ourselves and the universe. Life itself is celebration. It is celebration in the divine fellowship of all beings. Celebrating the community of kindred hearts and souls brings us joy and renews our spirit of life and hope for the future.

Wherein lies happiness? In that which becks
our ready minds to fellowship divine,
a fellowship with essence.
-John Keats

+++ WE ARE ONE +++

We are one humanity
on this spaceship Earth
with common hopes and aspirations.

We are one family
on this global lifeboat
struggling to stay afloat

We are one people
capable of horrible self-destruction
or creating a new and peaceful world.

We are one body
inseparably intertwined
in both life and death.

We are one mind
searching for itself
through time and space

We are one spirit
of vital stardust
evolving toward its destiny.

- A Personal Survey -

This is the time to stop and reflect on your life and celebration of community by completing the following sentences as rapidly as you can. Express the first thought or feeling that comes to mind. Make additional comments as needed.

1. In my community -

2. I can help improve my neighborhood -

3. One of the best things I can do for the global community is -

4. My friends -

5. The way I really like to be treated is -

6. I could volunteer to serve -

7. Our laws could be improved -

8. I especially enjoy celebrating with others during -

9. Sometimes it is difficult to empathize with -

10. A reward of unselfishness is -

15

- HUMAN SPIRITUAL EVOLUTION -

The greater part of progress is the desire to progress.
-Seneca

Life is a comic-tragic opera of struggle and adaptation to constant changes in our global environment. Physical and spiritual evolution is the consumation of eons of growth and variation. But with the emergence of human consciousness and creative powers, continued progress and evolution is increasingly centered in the desires of our own hearts and minds. Unfortunately, man's history is largely a disturbing record of incessant war against others and his own self.

As humankind prepares to move into the twenty-first century, it must learn to cope more adequately with problems threatening its very existence. Indeed, human history is largely a record of interpersonal strife over power, material resources and dogmatic disputes. But we also have a distinctive record of progressive exploration and unique creativity in such things as art, music, science and technology, which have greatly enriched our lives.

Most cultures have expressed these evolutionary struggles in creation stories and legends of heroes who have successfully overcome the many obstacles to survival. These great legends portray human progress as significant steps in spirtual growth and development - especially in the use of newly acquired knowledge to successfully understand and control the powerful forces within us and the world in which we live.

Indeed, since human creation, our spiritual evolution has been an ongoing struggle between positive life-enhancing predispositions and our more destructive and negative inclinations. Continual religious intolerance, persecution, inquisition and wars have continued to restrict many forms of spiritual expression.

Nature knows no pause in progress and development.
He who moves not forward goes backward.
Progress has not followed a straight line but a spiral
with rhythms of progress and retrogression,
of evolution and dissolution.
-Johann Wolfgang von Goethe

Positive spiritual development has been a slow process. The early Babylonians and many other cultural groups believed that human destructive forces were the result of evil spirits possessing the body which had to be properly exorcised and controlled. Egyptian culture professed that humans had a soul ("Ka") that functioned as a unique spirit of higher intelligence which guided us in this life and the next. Hinduism recognized a personal soul ("Atman") as having transcendental powers for eventually uniting with the universal spiritual reality, God (or "Brahman"), through a gradual process of ethical human development and compensation ("Karma"). Then the Greek philosophers began to refine the spiritual concept of one creative power ("monism") and early scientific ideas of universal cosmic energy.

Everything originates in a whirl of being and becoming,
out of previous states of existence.
In that one desire stirred into being,
desire that was the earliest seed of Spirit.
- Hindu Rig-Veda

All cultures have sought to personify the forces of good and evil in a hierarchy of deities. For example, some of the more commonly known Roman gods and their human attributes include Venus (beauty and desire) and her son Cupid (love), Mars (war), Bacchus (wine and revelry) and Psyche (soul and immortality). Mythological stories portray these gods as highly influential in human life, such as the marriage of Cupid and Psyche which produced the offspring of youth, pleasure and joy. Even today, some of these deities are recognized during holidays and special occasions, such as Mardi Gras.

Humans gradually began to develop stories of cultural heroes who performed unusual deeds with god-like spiritual powers and intervention. These spiritual journeys for self-realization and control have been portrayed in epic adventures of Gilgamesh, Horus, Krishna and numerous others. Many of these events were also incorporated in the legends of Biblical characters and real historical persons such as Buddha, Homer, Socrates and Jesus. Biblical stories dramatically portray the many difficulties in humankind's spiritual progress and development, beginning with its special creation and rapid downfall.

Specifically, according to Genesis, God said *let us make man in our image.* But apparently after some deliberation with the other powers that were available, he finally decided to create man in his own image. But then God realized that man needed a helpmate. So he took one of Adam's ribs and made it into the first woman, Eve. It is said that this is why women continue to rib men and confirms that God had a great sense of humor - as well as being pleased with his creation!

Then Eve successfully tempted Adam with the forbidden fruit of wisdom from the tree of knowledge that resulted in their expulsion from the Garden of Eden. Shortly thereafter, Adam and Eve gave birth to Cain and Abel and quickly became the first dysfunctional family, with intense sibling rivalry which culminated in the murder of Abel.

Cain was cursed by God and became a vagabond who finally dwelt in the strange land of Nod where he got a wife who was obviously an outsider with different genetic predispositions; this union resulted in another change in human evolution since their numerous progeny included other persons with similar homicidal inclinations.

Since the legendary downfall, mankind has been perceived as constantly struggling with the knowledge of good and evil and the problems of how to *wisely* control his deceitful and violent tendencies. Since early times, men continued to intermarry with strange "giants" (or Biblical Nephilim) which furthered human variation and wickedness.

Eventually, in many cultures, the gods then intervened with great floods and other disasters in attempts to exterminate violence and corruption from the earth and to begin anew with more righteous people. Even Zeus did not feel secure until he destroyed the vicious giants, known as "men of bronze", with a flood!

Let right deeds be thy nature, not the fruit that comes from them.
And live in action! Labor! Make those acts thy piety,
casting all self aside, concerning gain and merit...
Since in the performance of plain duty
man mounts to his highest bliss.
- Bhagavad Gita 2: 47-51

Thankfully, the story of Noah and the ark conveys hope of a new start for humankind. After the flood, Noah pleased God to the extent that even though he noted that man continued to have evil inclinations, the Lord vowed he would no longer kill every living creature as he had just done. Then he created the rainbow as a token of his covenant. The rainbow continues to be a univeral symbol of joyful hope and renewal for all who see it!

Since then, through thousands of years of trial and tribulation, many great spiritual guides and leaders, such as Buddha, Jesus and Ghandi, have attempted to show the way with compelling demonstrations of human brotherhood, love, compassion and self-control. As a result, considerable spirtual progress and insight have been acquired, but with questionable personal and societal results.

Now we have become consciously aware that our personal and social evolution, and the very future of the world in which we live, depends on the nurturance of spiritual progress and the sublimation of destructive tendencies. With the relatively recent development of modern technology, the dangers of self-extinction become increasingly apparent through threats of nuclear terror and proliferation, uncontrolled population growth, genocide and global pollution.

It now appears obvious that our fate depends on how *rapidly* we can progress in controlling our aggressive instincts toward violence, war and exploitation through education and cooperative endeavor. A great scientist, Erwin Schrodinger, said that every day of a person's life represents a small bit in the evolution of our species and that, while the raw material for this ongoing transformation is in our inheritable spontaneous genetic mutations, the *most decisive influenc*e is our own behavior and habits of life!

Accordingly we need to rededicate ourselves to the daily *practice* of self-respect, benevolence, good will and loving stewardship for all things. Only through such dedicated spiritual progress, can we contribute to positive human evolution and a brighter future.

- LET YOUR LIGHT SHINE -

You are the salt of the earth and the light of the world.
Let your light so shine before men
that they may see your good works,
and glorify your father which is in heaven.
- Jesus Christ

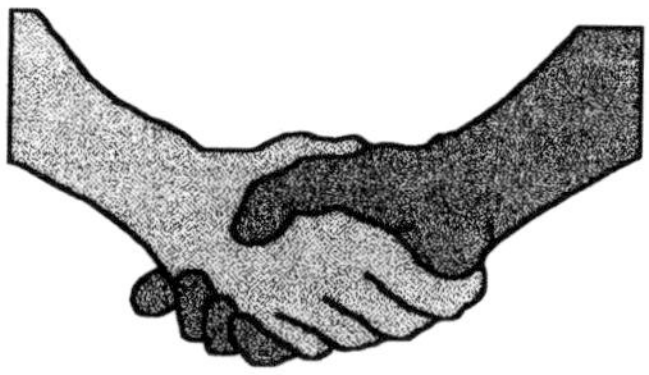

* PEACEFUL CONFLICT

Respect the right to disagree.

Express your real concerns.

Share common goals and interests.

Open yourself to different points of view.

Listen carefully to all proposals.

Understand the major issues involved.

Think about possible consequences.

Imagine several possible alternative solutions.

Offer some reasonable compromises.

Negotiate mutually fair cooperative agreements.

+++PROGRESS+++

My interest is in the future because I am going to spend the rest of my life there.
- C.F. Kettering

Millions long for immortality who do not know what to do with themselves on a rainy Sunday afternoon.
- Susan Ertz

The best thing about the future is that it comes only one day at a time.
- Anon

Progress is not an accident, but a necessity...it is part of nature.
- Herbert Spencer

"Be yourself" is about the worst advice you can give to some people.
- T.L. Masson

God help those who do not help themselves!
- Addison Mizner

I sing the progress of a deathless soul.
- John Milton

Spiritual thoughts are stronger than any material force - and rule the world.
- Ralph Waldo Emerson

A guilty conscience is the mother of invention.
- Carolyn Wells

All progress has been from people who took unpopular positions.
- Adlai Stevenson

- A Personal Survey -

This is the time to stop and reflect on your life and spiritual evolution by completing the following sentences as rapidly as you can. Express the first thought or feeling that comes to mind. Make additional comments as needed.

1. What I have learned from history is -
2. Over the years I have become increasingly aware -
3. Good and evil -
4. Human knowledge -
5. Some powerful legends -
6. At times I have been at war with myself over -
7. When I see a rainbow -
8. Great creation myths -
9. Civilization progresses -
10. My spiritual evolution -

- REFLECTIONS -

- LOVE'S PHILOSOPHY -

The fountains mingle with the river,
and the rivers with the ocean;
The winds of heaven mix forever with a sweet emotion;
Nothing in the world is single;
All things by a law divine in one another's being mingle:
Why not I with thine?
-Percy Bysshe Shelley

*****

- PRAY -

Let us be at peace with our bodies and our minds.
Let us return to ourselves and become wholly ourselves.
Let us be aware of the source of being,
common to us all and to all living things.
Let us pray that we ourselves cease
to be the cause of suffering to each other.
-Thich Nhat Hanh

- BEAUTIFUL -

Beautiful faces are they that wear
The light of a pleasant spirit there;
Beautiful hands are they that do
Deeds that are noble, good and true;
Beautiful feet are they that go
Swiftly to lighten another's woe.
-McGuffey's Second Reader

*****

- IF I CAN STOP ONE HEART FROM BREAKING -

If I can stop one heart from breaking,
I shall not live in vain.
If I can ease one life the aching,
Or cool one pain,
Or help one fainting robin
Unto his nest again,
I shall not live in vain.
-Emily Dickinson

-THE GOOD SOUL-

The temperate soul is the good soul,
the soul which is in the opposite condition, that is, the foolish and intemperate, is the bad soul...
The temperate man, also just and courageous and holy,
cannot be other than a perfectly good man,
nor can the good man do otherwise than
well and perfectly whatever he does;
and he who does well must of necessity
be happy and blessed.

- Socrates

*****

- MORAL VIRTUE -

Moral virtue is a mean that lies between two vices,
one of excess and the other of deficiency,
and it aims at hitting the mean both
in feelings and in actions.
The mean is the most praiseworthy state.
But as a practical matter, we must sometimes aim a bit toward
excess and sometimes toward deficiency,
because this will be the easiest way of hitting the mean,
that is, what is right.

-Aristotle

- MAN'S TASK -

***Man's task is to become conscious of the contents
that press upwards from the unconscious.
His destiny is to create more and more consciousness.
As far as we can discern,
the sole purpose of human existence
is to kindle a light in the darkness of mere being.***
-Carl Jung

*****

- DESTINY -

***But all we find along our way
to times be-gone we owe,
The world is as it is today,
because men made it so.***

***And since today must be the sum
of all that went before,
Our lives may hold what is to come
when we shall be no more.***

***Now we are here and know not why,
the end, no man can say;
The answer to our lives may lie
long centuries away.***
-Edgar Guest

- THE HUMAN TOUCH -

'Tis the human touch in this world that counts,
the touch of your hand and mine,
Which means far more to the fainting heart
than shelter and bread and wine;
For shelter is gone when the night is o'er
and bread lasts only a day,
But the touch of the hand and the sound of the voice
sing on in the soul alway.
-Spencer Michael Free

*****

- PERSEVERANCE -

We must not hope to be mowers,
And to gather the ripe gold ears,
Unless we have first been sowers
And watered the furrows with tears.

It is not just as we take it,
This mystical world of ours,
Life's field will yield as we make it
A harvest of thorns or of flowers.
- Johann Wolfgang von Goethe

- DANCE OF THE ATOMS -

In the stillness I hear in every blade of grass,
In every speck of dust,
In every part of my own body,
In the visible and invisible worlds,
In the planets, the sun and the stars,
The joyous dance of the atoms
through endless time.
-Rabindrarath Tagore

*****

- GREAT CREATIVE SPIRIT -

The Creative Spirit is my guide -
I shall not want;
it gives me peace and restores my energy.
it leads me to do what is right.
Even though I will die I am not afraid
for it is in me and gives me comfort.
My Spirit provides for my needs
and gives me joy and delight.
Surely I shall be good and happy
as long as this Spirit is within me.

- YOUR PLACE -

Whoever you are, no matter how lonely,
the world offers itself to your imagination,
calls to you like the wild geese, harsh and exciting -
over and over announcing
your place in the family of things.
-Mary Oliver

*****

- SHARING -

Love cannot remain by itself - it has no meaning.
Love has to be put into action and that action is service.
Whatever form we are,
able or disabled,
rich or poor,
it is not how much we do,
but how much love we put into the doing
- a lifelong sharing of love with others.
-Mother Teresa

- SELF STUDY -

No one ever told us we had to study our lives, make of our lives a study, as in learning natural history or music, that we should begin with the simple exercises and then go on to the hard ones, practicing till strength and accuracy become one with the daring to leap into transcendence.

-Adrienne Rich

*****

- I AM -

I am myself
I live and breathe
I think and feel
I love and care
I hope and fear
I grow and change
I am forever becoming
me.

- GOD LIVES IN ALL -

Why do you go to the forest in search of the divine?
God lives in all, and abides with you too.
As fragrance dwells in a flower,
or reflection in a mirror,
so the Divine dwells inside everything;
seek therefore in your own heart.
-Tegh Bahadur

*****

- GOD'S WORLD -

O World, I cannot hold thee close enough!
Thy winds, thy wide gray skies!
Thy mists that roll and rise!
Thy woods, this autumn day,
that ache and sag and all but cry with color!
That gaunt crag to crush!
To lift the lean of that black bluff!
World, World, I cannot get thee close enough!
-Edna St. Vincent Millay

- *OPPORTUNITY -

Everyday is a wonderful
opportunity
to love, to learn, to laugh,
to care, to contribute,
and to
CELEBRATE
the
JOY of LIFE!

*****

- *HEART -

The Human heart
feels ***things***
the eyes cannot see,
and knows
what the mind
cannot understand!

- PEACE -

Lord, make me an instrument of thy peace.
Where there is hatred, let me sow love.
Where there is injury, pardon.
Where there is doubt, faith.
Where there is despair, hope.
Where there is darkness, light.
And where there is sadness, joy.

O, Divine Master,
grant that I may not so much seek
to be consoled, as to console;
to be understood, as to understand;
to be loved, as to love;
for it is in giving that we receive,
it is in pardoning that we are pardoned,
and it is in dying that we are born to eternal life.
-St. Francis of Assisi

-SUGGESTED READINGS-

Achterburg, Jeanne. *Imagery in Healing.* NY: New Science, 1986.
Borysenko, Joan and Miroslav Borysenko. *The Power of the Mind to Heal.* Carson, CA: Hay House, 1994.
Bucke, Richard Maurice. *Cosmic Consciousness.* NY: E.P. Dutton, 1969.
Capra, Fritjof. *The Tao of Physics.* NY: Bantam, 1976.
Cousins, Norman. *Head First- The Biology of Hope.* NY: E.P. Dutton, 1989.
Davies, Paul. *The Mind of God.* NY: Simon and Schuster, 1992.
Dossey, Larry. *Rediscovering the Soul.* NY: Bantam, 1989.
Dreher, Diane. *The Tao of Inner Peace.* NY: Harper, 1990.
Eiseley, Loren. *The Star Thrower.* NY: Times Books, 1978.
Emerson, Ralph Waldo. *Emerson's Essays.* NY: Harper & Rowe, 1951.
Franklin, Benjamin. *Poor Richard's Almanacks.* NY: Heritage Press, 1964.
Goleman, Daniel and Daniel Gurin (Eds.) *Mind Body Medicine.* NY: Consumers Reports Books, 1993.
Hanh, Thich Nhat. *The Miracle of Mindfulness.* Boston: Beacon Press, 1976.
Herbert, Nick. *Elemental Mind.* NY: Dutton, 1993.
Huxley, Aldous. *The Perennial Philosophy.* NY: Harper & Row, 1944.
Jefferson, Thomas, *The Life and Morals of Jesus of Nazareth.* NY: Beacon, 1951.
Joint Committee on the New Translation. *The New English Bible with the Apocrypha.* Oxford & Cambridge University Press, 1970.
Jung, C.G. *Psychological Reflections (Edited by Jolande Jacobi and R.F.C. Hull).* NJ: Princeton University Press, 1970.
Locke, Stephen and Douglas Colligan. *The Healer Within.* NY: E.P. Dutton, 1986.
Mansfield, Victor. *Synchronicity, Science and Soul-Making.* Chicago, Il: Open Court, 1995.
Maslow, Abraham H. *The Farther Reaches of Human Nature.* NY: Viking, 1971.
May, Rollo. *Man's Search For Himself.* London: George Allen & Unwin Ltd., 1953.
Misglove, Jeffrey. *The Roots of Consciousness.* Tulsa, OK: Council Oak Books, 1993.
Moore, Thomas. *Care of the Soul.* NY: Harper, 1992.
Myers, David G. *The Pursuit of Happiness.* NY: Avon, 1990.
Naparstek, Belleruth. *Staying Well with Guided Imagery.* NY: Warner, 1994.
Peale, Norman Vincent. *Dynamic Imaging.* Old Tappan, NJ: Sleming Revell, 1982.
Radhakrishnan, S. *The Bhagavad-Gita.* NY: Harper Torchbooks, 1948.
Valett, Robert E. *Self-Actualization.* Niles, IL: Argus Communications, 1974.
Whitman, Walt. *The Illustrated Leaves of Grass.* NY: Grosset & Dunlap, 1971.
Wordsworth, William. *Poems, Lyrics & Sonnets.* Mount Vernon, NY: Peter Pauper Press. Undated.

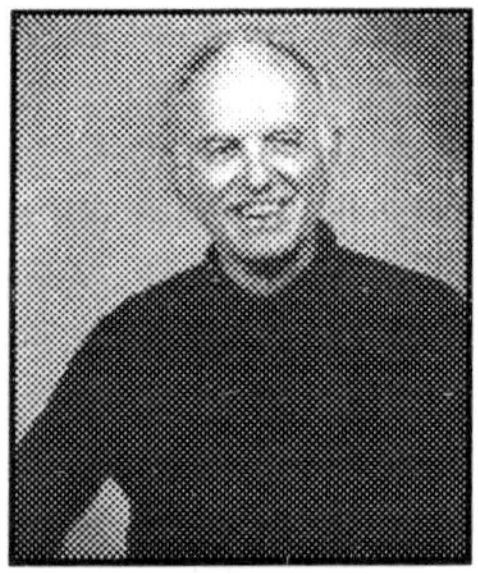

-About the Author-

Dr. Robert E. Valett received graduate degrees from the University of Chicago (M.A.) and the University of California at Los Angeles (Ed.D) with doctoral concentration in counseling and educational psychology. He taught psychology at Orange Coast College and the University of Canterbury in New Zealand and has worked as a licensed psychologist and special educator in public schools, clinics and private practice. As the author of many articles, books, motivational posters and materials on self-actualization, humanistic education, learning and behavior disorders, he has consulted and lectured throughout the United States and abroad. Dr. Valett is a recipient of the distinguished psychologist award from the San Joaquin Psychological Association and is a past president of the California Association of School Psychologists. He is a professor emeritus at California State University, Fresno, and remains creatively engaged with a scintillating wife, five children, grandchildren, workshops and community affairs. Please send comments, suggestions or requests for further information on *Spiritual Guides to Holistic Health and Happiness* directly to him at 5308 N. Colonial #102, Fresno, California 93704. E-Mail: robertv@csufresno.edu

OTHER WORKS BY DR. ROBERT E. VALETT

Self-Actualization
Humanistic Education
Getting It All Together
The Remediation of Learning Disabilities
Love and TLC
Dyslexia
Modifying Children's Behavior
The Psychoeducational Treatment of Hyperactive Children
Programming Learning Disabilities
The Practice of School Psychology
Effective Teaching
Developing Cognitive Abilities
100+ Peace Strategies

The ABC's of Happiness
Self-Affirmations
Peaceful Conflict Resolution

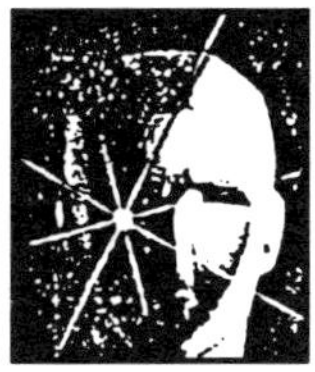

SPIRITUAL GUIDES

to

HOLISTIC HEALTH AND HAPPINESS

by Robert E. Valett

ISBN 0-938911-11-2

All profits from sales of this book are donated to charitable community groups. Quantity discounts can be obtained on bulk purchases by schools, churches, holistic health centers, clinics, and other non-profit organizations and workshops.

For additional copies of this book check your local book store or order directly from the distributor using the form below.

-SPECIAL ORDER FORM-

For each copy of SPIRITUAL GUIDES TO HOLISTIC HEALTH AND HAPPINESS by Robert E. Valett enclose a check for $12.95 plus $1.00 California tax and $3.00 for shipping and handling (add $1.00 for each additional book). Price is reduced 40% when ordering four or more copies.

To: American West Books
950 N. Van Ness Ave.
Fresno, CA 93726

Telephone 1-800-497-4909
Fax (209) 494-9266

Please send me _____ copies of this book as soon as possible.
Enclosed is my check for the amount of ________.

Name (please print) ______________________________

Address ______________________________

City ______________ **State** ____________ **Zip** ____________